ALKALINE DIET

THE MOST COMPLETE GUIDE TO CLEANSE YOUR BODY

DR. JOHN SLOAN

Table of Contents

Introduction

The importance of the body's acid–alkaline balance to overall health is being recognized by an increasing number of patients and therapists. In my book *L'équilibre acido-basique* (Geneva: Editions Jouvence, 1991), I explained what this balance is and how to correct it when it is lost in order to restore good health.

Experience has shown the need for a more detailed examination of certain points to make this corrective therapy easier to implement for the reader, including how to interpret urine pH measurements, choose corrective foods, create alkaline menus, decide dosages for alkaline supplements, and so forth.

The purpose of *The Acid–Alkaline Diet for Optimum Health* is to shed new light where needed. In this respect it is an eminently practical book. While it will stand perfectly well on its own, it also makes the ideal complement to *L'équilibre acido-basique*.

This book consists of three parts, each corresponding to one of the major questions about acid–alkaline balance.

1. How do I know if I have an acid problem?

Following a brief definition of the acidity problem, part one explains what tests are available, how to perform them, and, most importantly, how to interpret them.

2. How do I lower acidity through diet?

Diet plays a fundamental role in acid–alkaline balance. Part two provides detailed lists of foods that are alkalizing, foods that are acidifying, and weak-acid foods; a classification of foods according to their acidifying properties; guidelines for a balanced diet; an analysis of currently popular but acidifying meals; and numerous suggestions for alkaline-based menus.

3. How do I neutralize and eliminate acids?

Treatments using alkaline supplements—which are often applied incorrectly— are explained in part three in detail: dosages, how long a treatment should last, how to monitor the effectiveness of a supplement, what products are available, and so forth. Also explained is how to drain acids from the body and rejuvenate it with alkaline energy boosters.

By following the guidelines offered in this book, readers affected by acid problems will be working actively toward the recovery of their good health. I wish you every success.

Note: The fresh cheese called for in this book can be any of a large number of cheeses that have not been ripened and thus are intended for immediate consumption. American cottage cheese is on this list, as are ricotta, mozzarella, quark, fromage blanc, neufchâtel, and queso blanco. Especially prevalent in the recommendations in this book is fromage blanc for its spreadability; its consistency is also good for mixing with fruits and preserves. Fromage blanc is now available in many health food stores and supermarkets. Good substitutes for fromage blanc are fresh goat cheese, neufchâtel, and soft cream cheese, preferably the low-fat variety.

Cheeses and dairy foods that have a higher whey content will become more acidic as they age—this is why cottage cheese can be found listed as both an alkaline and an acid food. Generally the firmer large-curd cottage cheese will be more alkaline. Consumers should also be aware of the expiration date on the container, as the acidity of cottage cheese increases with age.

Part One

DEFINING ACIDITY

1

What Is Acid–Alkaline Balance?

The substances the body uses for building and functioning are quite numerous: there are approximately twenty amino acids, several dozen sugars and fatty acids, approximately forty vitamins, and one hundred or so minerals and trace elements. Each of these substances plays one or several specific roles in the body.

Despite the extreme diversity of these substances, it is possible to classify them in two major groups: basic (or alkaline) substances and acid substances. These two different groups of substances have opposing but complementary characteristics. To be healthy, the body needs both. When alkalines and acids are present in equal quantities, the acid–alkaline balance is achieved.

Many organic balances are necessary for good health: those between activity and rest, inhalation and exhalation, venous and arterial blood, energy intake and expenditure, and the production and elimination of toxins. Just as it is detrimental to disturb any one of these balances—for example, to eat more than the body needs or not rest enough to make up for daily activity—an excess of either acid or alkaline substances is very harmful to health.

WHAT IS AN ACID?

If you have ever bitten into a lemon or eaten rhubarb you know the most obvious characteristic of an acid: its taste. But acidic foods also stimulate salivation to dilute the acid, which brings out another property of acids—their harsh, even corrosive, nature.

We take advantage of this latter property in everyday life in many ways. Vinegar dissolves the calcium deposits that can form in pots and sinks, and some of today's cleaning products partially owe their cleansing qualities to the acids they contain. The corrosive nature of acids is also demonstrated by the well-known experiment of soaking a piece of meat or a coin in a cola-based beverage. After several days the meat will have dissolved totally and the surface of the coin will be scarred and pitted.

Chemically, acids are defined as substances that release hydrogen ions when dissolved in water. Some acids give off more hydrogen ions than others. Rhubarb and lemons, for example, are much more acidic than strawberries or tomatoes, which are also acidic foods.

Taste is not an infallible means for determining that a food is acidic, because acids can be partially neutralized and their taste obscured by the presence of other substances. Meat and cereal grains are not acidic to the taste, but they are very acidifying foods.

The degree of acidity of a substance is measured by determining its pH (see "How Acidity Is Measured"). It is also possible to identify a food as acidic by analyzing its mineral content. In fact, minerals can be divided into the same two basic groups: acidic and alkaline. The principal acidic minerals are sulfur, chlorine, phosphorus, fluoride, iodine, and silicon.

When a substance contains more acidic than alkaline minerals it is said to be acidic. Accordingly, mineral waters, which contain both types of mineral, are said to be alkaline when alkaline minerals, such as calcium and magnesium, predominate and acidic when sulfur, chlorine, or carbon dioxide prevail. A food rich in phosphorus—hazelnuts, for example—is more acidic than one that contains less phosphorus, like almonds.

WHAT IS AN ALKALINE?

Unlike acidic substances, alkaline substances in solution with water give up few or no hydrogen ions. The fewer hydrogen ions they release the less acidic they are—or, in other words, the more alkaline.

Also unlike acids, alkaline elements have no corrosive properties. They are "gentle" substances. Whereas lemon juice causes a sharp burning sensation if applied to a cut, milk does not. Alkaline substances can counter problems caused by acids. Potato juice, for example, soothes the pains of an acid stomach, and milk in large quantities can be an effective method of neutralizing the corrosiveness of acidic poisons swallowed by accident.

Alkaline foods have little or no acidic taste. In the most-alkaline foods, such as bananas, almonds, and fresh milk, not even the slightest trace of an acidic taste can be detected.

Alkaline minerals include calcium, sodium, magnesium, cobalt, and copper. The body contains more calcium than any other mineral, more than two pounds on average, most of which is concentrated in the skeleton.

As with acids, flavor is not a sufficient criterion for determining whether a food is alkaline. Certain foods—for example, bread and white sugar—are not at all acidic to the taste, but they are not alkaline foods. The acids these foods contain are freed in the course of their digestion and utilization by the body.

HOW ACIDITY IS MEASURED

As the difference between acids and alkalines is based more or less on their ability to free hydrogen ions, the unit that measures the degree of acidity or

9

alkalinity of a substance is shorthand for the substance's potential (p) for freeing hydrogen (H) ions, or pH.

The pH measuring scale goes from 0 to 14. The number 7 indicates the ideal balance between acid and alkaline substances and is known as a neutral pH. The greater potential a substance has for freeing hydrogen ions, the smaller is its pH number. The acidity range is from 6 to 0, zero indicating a state of absolute acidity. Conversely, a more alkaline pH is indicated by a higher figure, from 8 to 14, the last figure representing a state of total alkalinity (meaning a state in which no hydrogen ions are freed).

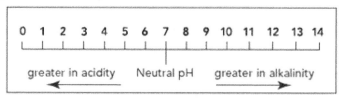

The pH scale

Note that on the pH measurement scale, the *greater* the degree of acidity, the *lower* the pH reading.

It is important to know that the transition from one figure to the next on this scale of measurement is not arithmetical but logarithmic, meaning that the values separating each unit are not of equal value along the scale but increase in proportion to their distance from the midway point of an even balance between acidity and alkalinity. The values are multiplied by 10 at each unit (see diagram "The pH scale"). In other words, if the concentration of hydrogen ions is 10 at a pH reading of 6, it will be 100 at a pH reading of 5; 1,000 at a pH reading of 4; 10,000 at a pH reading of 3; and so on. The gap between a pH of 6 and a pH of 5, for example, is not equal to the gap between a pH of 5 and a pH of 4; a gap of 90 in the first case becomes a gap of 900 in the second.

This means that the degree of acidity is much greater than one might think from the progression of the figures. Consequently, when urinary pH falls, for example, from 6 to 5, it is registering a much greater amount of acidification than that indicated by a decrease from 7 to 6.

The pH of different substances can be measured with a special reactive paper known as litmus paper. When put into contact with a dilution of the substance to be tested, the paper changes color to a degree that corresponds to the degree of acidity or alkalinity of that substance.

DIFFERENCE BETWEEN STRONG AND WEAK ACIDS

In addition to the degree of acidity as measured by the pH scale, acids can be characterized as either strong or weak. In fact, acids are rarely encountered in a free or isolated state; they are most often combined with an alkaline element. When the alkaline combined with the acid is strong (chemically speaking), the acid is of little consequence in the combination. The acid is called weak, as it is easy for the body to reject it. When the alkaline element is weak, however, the acid content is of much greater consequence. It is stable and mixes poorly with other elements, and it is referred to as strong.

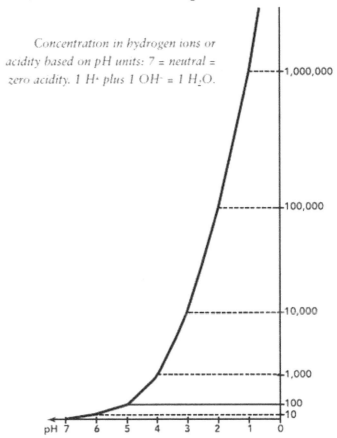

Concentration in hydrogen ions or acidity based on pH units: 7 = neutral = zero acidity. 1 H+ plus 1 OH- = 1 H₂O.

From the book *Terrain acidifié* by Jacques Fontaine (Geneva: Editions Jouvence, 1990).

Physiologically, strong acids—precisely because of their stability and resistance to combining—are much more difficult to neutralize and eliminate from the body than weak acids.

Strong acids come primarily from animal proteins. They chiefly consist of uric, sulfuric, and phosphoric acids. Their elimination from the body requires significant neutralization, a task performed by the liver as well as the normal elimination work of the kidneys. Because the kidneys can only eliminate a fixed amount of strong acids on a daily basis, however, any excess is stored in the tissues. Consequently, it is important to monitor the consumption of animal proteins.

Weak acids are primarily of plant origin (carbohydrates and vegetable proteins), except for those coming from yogurt and whey, which are of animal origin. Weak acids include citric, oxalic, pyruvic, and acetylsalicylic acids. Weak acids are also called volatile acids,[1] because once they have been oxidized they are eliminated by the lungs in the form of vapors and gases, both as breath moisture and as carbon dioxide (CO_2). Their elimination is relatively easy, and there are no limits on the quantity that can be expelled from the body by the kidneys, unlike nonvolatile strong acids. When the body needs to increase the elimination of volatile acids, it does so simply by increasing the rate of respiration. The amount of volatile acids that can be eliminated is limited only by how fast and how deeply a person is able to breathe.

pH AND HEALTH

The body functions at its best when the pH of its internal biochemical environment, measured as a whole, is equal to 7.39, meaning slightly alkaline. The normal range of this optimum pH is very small, from a slightly more acidic reading of 7.36 to a more alkaline reading of 7.42. A reading of anything higher or lower than these figures indicates acidosis (from 7.36 to 7) or alkalosis (7.42 to 7.8). If these limits are exceeded, the body can no longer function, and death results.

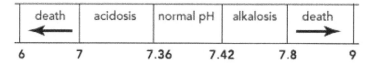

Fatal acidosis to fatal alkalosis

The zone of optimal health extends only from pH 7.36 to pH 7.42; illness will accompany any incidence of acidosis or alkalosis. Of these two, acidosis is by far the most common—more than half the population suffers from this condition. This is what we concentrate on in the remainder of the book.

The pH of the body's organic fluids and tissues varies from one part of the body to another. When we say the ideal pH of the body is 7.39, this refers primarily to the pH of the blood, and to a lesser extent that of the body's internal environment, meaning all organic fluids such as lymph and extra- and intracellular serums (fluids surrounding or within the cells). Blood is indeed "a very particular sap" (Goethe) whose pH must remain extremely stable to maintain the life of the physical organism. Even the slightest change of blood pH is rapidly corrected by the body, which restores it to the ideal measurement of 7.39. When the body is unable to perform this task, physical and mental disorders quickly appear.

The pH of the internal environment, the basic "ground" biochemical terrain, can tolerate more significant changes than that of the blood, but the pH of the internal environment should never go beyond 7.36 or 7.42 if good health is to be maintained.

Many individual organs and organic fluids, however, have a pH that is normally far above or below this ideal pH. The pH of urine, for example, may be 6, or even as low as 5 or 4.5. This is possible because urine is regularly eliminated and thus does not remain in the body for long. Areas of the body that are essentially acid include the small intestine (pH 6), the outer layers of the skin (pH 5.2), and the gastric region (pH 2). Others, in contrast, are quite alkaline: the inner layers of the skin (pH 7.35), the pancreatic juices (from pH 7.5 to pH 8.8), and the large intestine (pH 8).

These different values are all normal and correspond to precise needs of the body. For example, the extremely acidic nature of the gastric region is indispensable for protein digestion, and the high acidity of the skin helps it destroy microbes before they can enter the body.

So restoring the acid–alkaline balance does not mean bringing the gastric region's pH 2 up to pH 7—that would cause serious digestive problems—but rather restoring the pH of the basic internal biochemical terrain. The acidification of the internal terrain is in fact the source of all health troubles caused by acidity.

HOW THE BODY DEFENDS ITSELF AGAINST ACIDIFICATION

Whenever there is an imbalance between acid and alkaline substances, whether in the body's entire system or in a particular organ, the body is forced to react in self-defense. It has two means at its disposal to take action: to reduce the amount of the excessive substance by eliminating it from the body; and to partially neutralize the substance by forming neutral salts with the help of elements whose properties are the opposite of those causing the problem.

Let's examine the first of these solutions more closely.

The task of getting rid of excess acid in the body falls to the organs responsible for elimination: the lungs and kidneys.

The most rapid means for getting rid of a sudden intake of acids is via the respiratory system. By oxidizing acids, the lungs release them with each breath in the form of carbon dioxide and breath moisture. This is a fairly easy solution, as it simply requires increasing the volume and rate of the breath to intensify the pace of elimination and adapt it to the body's immediate physical needs.

Unfortunately, this method is capable of dealing only with weak acids. Fixed acids, which are nonvolatile and cannot be exhaled as a gas by the lungs, can be eliminated through the kidneys only, in a solid form. Uric, sulfuric, and similar acids must therefore be filtered out of the bloodstream by the kidneys and sent out of the body diluted in the urine. The kidneys, unlike the lungs, cannot adapt their elimination potential in accord with the needs of the body. Even working at maximum capacity, the kidneys cannot eliminate more than a certain daily fixed amount.

The accumulation of excess acid in the body's internal environment would be irremediable if there were no other exit available: the skin, specifically the sweat glands. Often the skin is overlooked as a means of elimination, but it is very useful for the disposal of acids.

Distributed over the entire surface of the skin, the sweat glands—of which there are more than 2 million—can expel strong acids because they work similarly to the kidneys and eliminate the same kind of wastes. Strong acids can be flushed from the body diluted in sweat, although in lesser quantities than in urine, as the body loses less than a quart of sweat a day compared to about one and a half quarts of urine. Furthermore, sweat carries a much smaller amount of toxins than does urine.

THE BUFFER SYSTEM

Acids and alkaline substances possess opposing characteristics. When they combine, their respective properties cancel each other out. This process is similar to what occurs whenever two opposites are brought together. If hot and cold, or black and white, are blended, their respective properties cancel each other out, and the result is a temperature that is neither hot nor cold but warm, or a color that is neither black nor white but gray.

The combination of an acid and an alkaline is designated in chemistry as a *neutral salt.* It is neutral because it possesses neither acidic nor alkaline properties.

1 acid + 1 alkaline = 1 neutral salt

A neutral salt no longer influences the solution it is in, such as blood or cellular serums. Neutralization of excess acids restores the acid–alkaline balance to the ideal pH of the internal environment, 7.39, which is itself almost neutral.

The alkaline substances the body uses to neutralize or buffer strong acids, or to counteract the sudden intake of a massive amount of weak acids, can be found throughout the body, not just in the blood. Alkaline substances in the bloodstream are utilized, but because blood pH can fluctuate only slightly, they

14

are only minimally drawn upon. Instead the body makes use of alkaline elements found in less important parts of the body, such as the tissues of the internal organs.

When this defense system is used only occasionally, the alkaline elements thus lost are easily replaced by the alkaline minerals found in food, and the tissues suffer no ill effects from making what amounts to a loan of their alkaline components. Problems occur, however, when the tissues are forced to relinquish their alkaline elements on a regular basis, every day or even several times a day. In this case the body's alkaline reserves inevitably gradually diminish. The word *reserves*, it should be noted, is something of a misnomer; these alkaline substances have not been set aside by the body for the express purpose of dealing with excess acid. These minerals are components of the tissues themselves and fulfill a very precise role in that regard.

Repeated withdrawals therefore create a shortage of alkaline minerals in these organic tissues. The critical mineral loss becomes even more pronounced when the plundering is intense and prolonged. Modern lifestyle and diet encourage such exploitation of the body's buffer system. It is the source of a host of troubles and diseases, as well as the general sense of malaise suffered by many in our contemporary civilization.

HOW ACIDIFICATION MAKES THE BODY SICK

When its internal environment becomes acidified, the body can fall ill in three different ways.

The first is connected to the activity of enzymes. Enzymes are the "worker drones" behind all the biochemical transformations that take place in the body and on which the proper functioning of the organs depends. Enzymes can perform their task correctly only in an environment with a clearly defined pH; otherwise their activity can be disrupted or even cease completely. When their activity is merely slowed down, illness appears. If there is a complete interruption, the body can no longer function, and death results. Before this extreme stage is reached, different ailments set in as an increasing number of enzymes find their world disturbed by the acidification of the internal environment.

The second way the body becomes ill is due to the harsh, corrosive nature of acids present in excess amounts within the tissues. Before they are neutralized by alkaline substances, the acids irritate the organ with which they come in contact. Inflammation, sometimes quite painful, results, as well as lesions or hardening of the tissues. This primarily affects the organs charged with the elimination of strong acids, such as the skin and kidneys. Many cases of eczema, hives, itching, and red patches on the skin are due to the irritation caused by excessively acidic sweat. The most susceptible regions are those where sweat has a tendency to collect: in the armpits, behind the knees, under the wristwatch band, or, in babies, under the diaper. When the urine is overloaded with acid, urination is painful and the urinary tract "burns," becoming inflamed (urethritis) or infected (cystitis).

Ailments triggered by harsh acid that are invisible to outsiders but are keenly felt by the victims include pains in the joints (arthritis), nerves (neuritis), and intestines (enteritis, colitis, and burning sensations in the anus).

The fragile state of the tissues resulting from the invasive presence of acid makes them vulnerable to microbial or viral infection as well. Lesions of the mucous membranes—such as in the respiratory system—allow easier penetration by and multiplication of microbes in the tissues. This is aggravated by the fact that the immune system's effectiveness can also be impaired by acid activity, which lowers the production and strength of the white blood cells responsible for attacking microbes.

The third cause of suffering from excess acid is loss of minerals, since the body gives up alkaline minerals to neutralize acids. This demineralization can be quite significant and can affect any organ because alkaline minerals are stored in all the body's tissues.

The best-known consequences of demineralization are problems affecting the skeleton and teeth. Bones lose their calcium, and along with it their resistance and flexibility, to the point where they break far too easily (for example, spontaneous hip fractures), lose their density (osteoporosis), become inflamed at the joints (rheumatism), wear away the intervertebral disks (sciatica), and so forth. Teeth can also become more brittle because of mineral loss. They can chip, become oversensitive to hot and cold foods, or become more susceptible to cavities.

The brittleness caused by demineralization also weakens hair, which loses its shine and resilience and starts falling out in greater quantity. Fingernails split and break under the slightest impact; skin dries and cracks or wrinkles; the gums become deformed and oversensitive and bleed easily.

ILLNESSES CAUSED BY ACIDIFICATION

Acidification engenders many afflictions that manifest in various ways. An individual suffering from excessive acid will not contract them all, only those that take advantage of the person's specific physiological weaknesses. Weak points are determined by temperament, heredity, accidents, lifestyle, and sometimes profession. With some people it is primarily the skin or respiratory system that is afflicted; with others it is the nerves or teeth, the gums, the eyes, or the spinal column.

Besides the illnesses listed above, acidification of the internal environment leads to great fatigue, even in the absence of any physical or mental effort. Generally the person afflicted no longer has any drive or enthusiasm, tires quickly, and takes a long time to recover from exertion. The individual tends to be touchy and irritable, to worry too much, and to sleep poorly, and may even become depressed. The noxious effect of acids on the nerves is easily explained: minerals like magnesium, calcium, and potassium that the nervous system needs to function properly are precisely the alkaline minerals the body takes away to neutralize acids.

Individuals suffering from acidification often are sensitive to the cold, have low blood pressure, and are subject to episodes of low blood sugar. All the functions of the endocrine glands tend to slow down, except for those of the thyroid gland, which become hyperactive. The immune system is weakened as well, and recurring infections of the respiratory tract (colds, laryngitis, flu, bronchitis) or urinary tract (cystitis) appear with distressing frequency because of both low immune response and the ease with which microbes can penetrate the body through tiny lesions in the mucous membranes of the respiratory and urinary tracts.

A surprising number and variety of physical problems and diseases can be caused by acidity. Indeed, a triple action can prompt their appearance: enzymatic disturbances, aggressive activity by acids, and demineralization are three factors capable of striking any organic tissue.

Of course, such problems are not always caused solely by acids. Bleeding gums, for example, can be the result of poor dental hygiene or a lack of vitamin C. But a person suffering from excessive acidity is often simultaneously or successively stricken by several of these afflictions. As varied as the conditions may appear, however, the remedy is always the same: the deacidification of the internal environment.

ACIDOSIS: A WIDESPREAD PROBLEM

Today the vast majority of the populace in Western (industrialized) nations suffers from problems caused by acidification, because both modern lifestyle and diet promote acidification of the body's internal environment.

In general, the current standard diet is primarily composed of acidic or acidifying elements (proteins, cereals, sugars). Alkaline foods such as vegetables are eaten in much smaller quantities; their alkaline content is insufficient to neutralize surplus acids. Furthermore, the consumption of stimulants like tobacco, coffee, tea, and alcohol—every one of which has an extremely acidifying effect on the body—has grown to enormous proportions.

Stress, nervous tension, noise, shortage of time, and other pressures are facts of life today and contribute to increasing the body's acidification through the physiological disturbances they create.

Physical exercise—which can play an important role in maintaining acid–alkaline balance—is more often than not either insufficient or excessive. In both cases, acidification of the body's internal environment is the result.

Of all the factors causing acidification, the most important is unquestionably food. The majority of acidosis sufferers can be treated simply by significantly reducing their consumption of acids and increasing their consumption of alkaline foods.

What Is a Metabolic Weakness Toward Acids?

There is a special category of individuals, however, who are sick not only because of an unhealthy lifestyle and an excessive intake of acids. They also suffer from a metabolic weakness that is particularly susceptible to acids.

Some illnesses arise because a person's body is unable to properly metabolize a particular nutrient. Partially or completely unmetabolized nutrients stagnate in the body, causing it to fall ill either through their own toxic effects or by disrupting the body's functioning. In diabetes, for example, the substance that is poorly metabolized is sugar; in rheumatism it is proteins; in obesity it is fat; in celiac disease it is gluten; and in water retention it is salt. These are just a few of the many substances, acids among them, that the body may have trouble metabolizing.

Difficulty metabolizing acids primarily involves weak acids. Weak acids are normally quite easy to oxidize, and their elimination through the lungs in the form of carbon dioxide or breath moisture makes the strong alkaline substances with which they were combined available for the body's use. As a rule, foods rich in weak acids, such as fruits, whey, yogurt, and vinegar, contribute a large number of alkaline elements to the body. But this is not always true for everyone, specifically that category of people whose metabolisms have trouble oxidizing weak acids.

For such people, acids are poorly oxidized, if at all, and they remain in the body without releasing the alkaline substances with which they are combined. In people with this metabolic weakness, foods that would normally contribute a high quota of alkaline substances instead have the effect of acidifying the internal environment. The same food can have an entirely different effect depending on the body of the person who ingests it. This is why some dietitians declare that lemon is an alkalizing food while others claim it is acidifying. Both are correct. The error lies in not determining whether the physical constitution of the person eating the food has an inherent metabolic weakness toward acids.

People afflicted with this metabolic debility must take additional precautions with their diets. It is essential that they carefully regulate the amount of foods they eat that are rich in weak acids (see the list "Weak-Acid Foods" in chapter 3).

Normally, this group of weak-acid foods doesn't figure in the classifications set up to help people maintain their acid–alkaline balance. Foods are generally divided into only two groups: acidifying and alkalizing. Weak-acid foods are usually included in the list of alkalizing foods, since with their weak acids they have an alkalizing effect on most people. But the lack of a third list of weak-acid foods could lead to serious problems for individuals whose Achilles' heel is metabolizing acids. They could consume large quantities of fruits, vinegar, and so on, confident they were alkalizing their internal environments, whereas in fact they would be creating precisely the opposite effect.

The problems caused by acidification should not be treated individually, but as a whole. Because acidification of the internal environment is responsible for so many different symptoms and illnesses, the most effective treatment for these conditions is to reduce or eliminate acidification. This is the surest way to make all the problems it has caused disappear.

Simple treatment of surface symptoms may bring relief, but it provides very little in the way of long-term effects because the fundamental imbalance in the body's internal environment remains unchanged. Treating only the symptoms forces the sufferer to run from one specialist to another, spending the morning at the dermatologist's getting treatment for eczema, then dividing the afternoon between the rheumatologist for painful joints and the dentist for gum problems. In contrast, focusing treatment on the main problem—reversing the acidification of the body's internal environment—goes to work right at the root of these ailments and treats them all.

The treatment plan to counter acidification aims first to reduce the amount of acids the body takes in. This is an indispensable step; as long as large quantities of acids are entering the body, all other measures have only a temporary palliative effect. Diet is adjusted so that alkaline foods and drinks predominate over acid foods. Dietary reform is a simple step, but its effect is considerable. Improved oxidation of acids is obtained by introducing or increasing physical activity (walking, sports). Eliminating the acids already present in the tissues is accelerated by consuming medicinal plants that increase the flow of urine (diuretics) and those that enhance the production of sweat (sudorifics).

An additional measure, which has proven to be indispensable in the majority of cases, is to take alkaline mineral supplements, not only to help the body eliminate the acids ingested during the day but also, and more importantly, to facilitate elimination of the acids lodged in the deep tissues of the body. This is a fundamental step, because the body is extremely reluctant to take acids embedded in the tissues back into the bloodstream where they can be transported to the lungs, kidneys, and skin for elimination. The return of acids to the blood carries a serious risk of dangerously altering its pH. To protect the blood, the body tends to let these acids remain in the tissues. However, a significant introduction of alkaline elements into the body allows the acids to be eliminated, for these alkaline substances act as a buffer and let the acids make their way back to the surface in the form of neutral salts. In this form they can cause no harm to the blood pH.

The various measures that can be taken to deacidify the body's internal environment (explained at length in parts two and three) cause all the acids embedded in the deep tissues to gradually resurface and be eliminated. Over time this cleansing leads to a profound deacidification of the body, which not only treats the sufferer but protects him or her from any recurrence of the problem.

2

Detecting Acidification

How can you tell if you are suffering from acidification? There are several tests that are easy to perform and interpret. The most important is also the most common, the test that measures urinary pH. Most often, however, you need to have the results of this test confirmed by another test.

Although two tests performed in a complementary way are enough for a professional to determine whether your internal environment is acidic, it is interesting to perform them all, because each reveals another aspect of your physiology, especially with regard to the elements that come into play to make the body acidic.

TEST 1: ANALYSIS OF URINARY pH

As noted, the test for determining the pH of the urine is simple to perform and gives fairly significant information on the degree of acidification from which you may be suffering. It consists of measuring the pH of the urine with litmus paper, which is a paper specially manufactured to make this kind of measurement.

To maintain good health the body is constantly seeking to get rid of the excess acids that irritate the tissues and deplete them of minerals. One of the principal exits it uses for this purpose is the renal system (kidneys). The normal rate of acid excretion through the kidneys gives urine a pH that falls between 7 and 7.5. By testing the degree of acidity of the urine, you can determine whether your body is rejecting a normal quantity of acids. If the excretion rate is higher than normal, the urinary pH will also be more acid, the sign of an overflow of acids that the body is attempting to get rid of. But this overflow is also an indication that the body is saturated and therefore in an acid state, with all the detriments that this can have on your health.

There is thus a close correspondence between the acid pH of the body's internal environment and that of the urine: urine becomes acidic when the body's internal environment becomes acidic. But the value of this test does not stop there. As we will see later in this section, charting how and when urinary pH is either neutral or alkaline yields other valuable information on the state of the internal environment and the way the body is metabolizing acids.

Necessary Materials

To measure urinary pH, all you need is litmus paper, which can be purchased in drugstores, pharmacies, and some health food stores.

Litmus paper has properties that cause it to change color when it comes in contact with acidic or alkaline substances. The color it changes to when in contact with a substance tells you whether the substance is acid or alkaline. It even indicates the strength of the acidity or alkalinity of a substance because the color change becomes more intense if a substance exhibits an extreme pH.

Litmus paper gets its name from the Scandinavian word for certain mosses and lichens that provide the dye that gives the paper its color. This coloring material turns red in acid solutions and blue in alkaline solutions. The neutral blue-violet dye usually comes from a plant in the Euphorbiacea family, such as the croton, though Mediterranean lichens are also often used.

The different shades of color that the coloring agent adopts allow the degree of a substance's acidity or alkalinity to be measured. Each shade of color corresponds to a precise pH value. The value is not indicated on the litmus paper itself, however, but on a color chart that comes with the paper. This chart includes every shade of color the litmus paper can adopt, with its corresponding pH value next to it.

The most common litmus papers available allow pH measurements between 4.5 and 9 to be taken; others have a narrower range of between 5.2 and 7.4. The clearly visible changes from one shade to the next are provided either in half units, which results in a scale that runs 4.5–5.0–5.5–6.0, and so on; or in measurements from 0.2 to 0.4, for example 5.3–5.5–5.8–6.2, and so on. Both systems are sufficiently precise for testing urinary pH.

A large variety of litmus papers is available. In pharmacies and drugstores you can buy the Neutralit Merck or Ames brands and through the internet the pH stixs of pHion Nutrition, which give indications in small .25 unit increments. Several other brands are packaged with alkaline mineral supplements that are sold commercially for the purpose of correcting the pH of the internal environment (for more on these see chapter 7).

The paper is sold in rolls from which pieces can be torn as needed, in small rectangular packets that are precut to the desired size, or even as small rods on which this reactive paper has been glued.

The shades of the colors vary according to manufacturer. Some papers go from yellow to blue, others from yellow to red. The transition from one shade of color to the next is obvious enough on any one of these papers to avoid any possibility of confusion. Some brands offer rods on which three different shades of colors are displayed simultaneously in order to make reading them easier.

How to Proceed

22

Litmus paper needs to be put in contact with the substance to be tested. The most simple method consists of holding the paper in the flow of urine for one or two seconds, just long enough to moisten it. The acid of the urine reacts with the paper, causing it to change color. The paper is then matched to the indicator scale on the color chart. The figure of the corresponding urinary pH is located right next to the color. Remember that it is neutral at 7; at 6.5 and under it is acid; and at 7.5 and above it is alkaline.

A single measurement is not enough to draw any valid conclusions about the state of the internal environment; pH can vary at different times of the day because of activity, meals, physical effort, stress, and so forth. To be truly representative, the measurements must be taken several times a day for four to five days in succession. You should note the data collected from these readings on a chart (see diagram "Urinary pH Record") to obtain an overall picture of pH over time.

As a rule, the first urination in the morning is not representative of your normal pH because it contains all the acids filtered by the kidneys that have accumulated overnight. The first test should therefore be made with the second urination of the morning. The second test should be made on the urine before lunch, and the third before the evening meal. It is very important to take the test before the meal, because the pH can temporarily vary significantly depending on what beverages and foods you have consumed. Besides these three tests, you may measure and note urine pH at other times of the day just as complementary data.

The chart on which the measurements of urine pH are listed consists of five columns, as shown in the example below.

URINARY pH RECORD

Date	Morning	Noon	Evening	Observations
6.1.06	7	7.5	7	had dinner at a restaurant
6.2.06	5	6.5	6.5	
6.3.06	7	7.5	6	stressful afternoon at work
6.4.06	7	7.5	7	

The first column is for the dates on which you take the measurements. The three following columns are for the morning, noon, and evening readings (from urinating before the meal). The fifth column is for recording potentially significant events that may have influenced the pH value—for example, an especially large meal or one that differs from your usual fare, a meal at a restaurant, alcohol consumption, an extra workload, playing sports, a significant amount of stress, or other various tensions. Be aware that the effects of events such as these on urinary pH do not always appear on the same day the events occurred but sometimes on the following day, when one or two pH readings may differ from their norms.

You can easily draw such a chart yourself, but a ready-to-use chart is included on page 196 for you to photocopy so you always have a clean copy for reference.

After a week or two there will be enough data to reveal a predominant pH value for each day, as well as for each segment of the day. Except for variations that are due to changes from your habitual activity or other significant incidents, these values should remain relatively constant over time.

How to Interpret the Results

Readings of urinary pH can have only three possible results: under 7, between 7 and 7.5, and above 7.5. While the interpretation of a pH below 7 is a simple matter, because it always indicates that the individual's internal environment has become acidified, this is not the case with the other two possible readings, which require a small additional analysis.

pH below 7 (Indicative of an Acid pH)

A pH in this range testifies to acidic urine. Regular readings indicating acidic urine are an unmistakable revelation that the body's internal environment is also acidic. This acidification is more significant if the reading is low. A reading of 6 or 6.5 indicates that there is only a slight degree of acidification, but the internal environment is extremely acidic if the urinary acid gives a reading of 5 or 4.5. Anyone obtaining consistent readings in this latter range is strongly advised to adopt without delay the methods for removing acid from the body discussed in parts two and three of this book.

pH between 7 and 7.5 (Indicative of a Neutral pH)

This is the normal pH of a person in good health and is what you are aiming for. A reading in this range indicates a good acid–alkaline balance *as long as the first urination of the day is acidic*, reflecting all the accumulated acids eliminated by the body during the night. If the first urine is not acidic it is a sign that acids are remaining in the body because the kidneys are not flushing them out properly. This means the internal environment is acidified even if urinary pH readings taken at other times of the day are neutral. Other tests involving foods and symptoms, discussed later in this chapter, can confirm this.

If your first urination of the day is neutral rather than acidic, you are suffering from acidification and should apply the necessary measures to address this problem, with a particular emphasis on the elimination of acids by the skin and kidneys. In fact, in this case an important piece of the problem resides in the eliminatory weakness of these organs.

pH above 7.5 (Indicative of an Alkaline pH)

As with a neutral pH, there are subtle issues to be considered in interpreting urine pH readings that are consistently above 7.5. There are three possibilities.

First, the internal environment has a good acid–alkaline balance or is slightly alkaline. Generally speaking, this is the case when the food eaten is particularly alkalizing, as is the case with some vegetarians who eat only small quantities of grains and dairy products. Such a reading may also be found for a person who takes alkaline mineral supplements on a daily basis when the body either does not need them or does not need so much of them.

INTERPRETING URINARY pH READINGS

pH	Urine quality	Internal environment quality	Note	Steps to take
below 7	acid	acid	acidifying lifestyle, or metabolism that has trouble with acids	deacidify the body
between 7 and 7.5	neutral	neutral	good health if first urination of the day is acid	maintain current hygiene
		acid	if first urination of the day is also neutral, metabolic inability to handle acids	deacidify internal environment, stimulate kidneys and skin
over 7.5	alkaline	alkaline	vegetarian diet or excessive use of alkaline mineral supplements	maintain current hygiene but avoid protein deficiency reduce intake of alkaline minerals
		acid	metabolic inability to handle acids	deacidify internal environment

These specific situations do not signify an imbalance or disease, but some precautions should be taken. Vegetarians must be careful to avoid deficiencies in their diets, especially of proteins. Those taking alkaline supplements should reduce their intake to a level that makes the pH of the urine neutral. (For more on this topic see chapter 7.)

Second, people who have a urinary pH clearly above 7.5 may be suffering from a glandular problem (adrenal or parathyroid glands) or other specific illnesses. These cases are extremely rare, and the people involved are generally already following a medical treatment plan for the problems caused by this imbalance.

The third possibility is the most likely: the urine is alkaline but the internal environment, paradoxically, is acidic. In this case the alkaline pH of the urine is not due to excessive intake of alkaline elements through diet (which the body attempts to get rid of, just as it does with excess acids), but to disproportionate withdrawal of alkaline substances from the organic tissues to neutralize heavy acidification of the internal environment.

This is common among people whose metabolism has difficulty digesting acids. Because the acids are poorly oxidized, they cannot leave the body through the respiratory system. The kidneys must pick up the slack and do double duty of elimination. Although these are the acids classified as weak, their accumulation is dangerous for the body, which will take extreme efforts to buffer itself against the avalanche of acids confronting it. This levy results in bringing a large quantity of alkaline elements into the urine and thus alkalizing it.

The urine is therefore alkaline not because of a net physiological gain in the quantity of alkaline substances, but because of a massive loss of alkaline elements due to the body's plunder of its reserves. This can easily be confirmed by analyzing the types of conditions a person in this situation suffers from to see whether they are among those caused by acidification. In this case it is extremely important to make the internal environment less acidic despite the alkalinity of the urine.

If the pH readings are not uniform during the course of the day, as in the cases mentioned above, but their variations occur regularly at specific times—for example, the urinary pH is acidic in the evening but neutral the rest of the day (except for the first urination of the morning), or vice versa—this indicates an excess of acidity in the internal environment and signals the necessity for restoring it to a neutral state.

TEST 2: ANALYSIS OF SYMPTOMS

Acid aggression on the tissues and the plundering of the body's reserves of alkaline minerals cause characteristic problems. One of the means used for determining whether a person's internal environment is acidified involves analyzing whether any problems he or she is suffering from currently, as well as any that were present in the past, are characteristic of those that accompany acidification.

The list below starts with the description of general symptoms and continues with ailments classified according to the parts of the body they affect.

If you are suffering from only one or two of the problems cited, your internal environment most likely is not acidified; or, if it is, the other characteristic problems have yet to manifest. To learn more you need to perform a test of urinary pH.

Of course, if you are afflicted with acidification you will not suffer from all the problems on the list. When reading the descriptions of these different problems, you may recognize some as conditions you had in the past and others as those you are currently dealing with. You may also recognize some as conditions to which you are susceptible even though you are not currently suffering from their full-blown versions. For example, you might have a tendency toward dry skin or joint pains without actually having eczema or rheumatism.

OVERALL STATE OF HEALTH

- Lack of energy: constant fatigue, loss of physical tone and psychic drive, decreasing activity, tires easily, difficulty in recovering strength following physical or mental effort, sensation of heaviness in the limbs, frequent and sudden feelings of inability to cope, sudden loss of energy following the consumption of acid foods
- Lower body temperature: sensations of intense and deep inner chills, frequently feels cold
- Weight loss specifically due to the decalcification of the bones
- Tendency to get infections because of decreased effectiveness of the body's defenses

MENTAL CONDITION

- Loss of drive, joy, and enthusiasm
- Sadness, dark thoughts, depressive tendencies
- High irritability
- Nervousness: agitation without cause, hyperactivity, sensitivity to high-pitched noises and often startled by them, easily stressed, difficulty dealing with stress

HEAD

- Very pale face (due to capillary contraction)
- Headaches
- Eyes tear easily and are sensitive (to cold, smoke, etc.)
- Conjunctivitis
- Inflammation of the corneas and eyelids

MOUTH

- Acidic saliva
- Loose teeth
- Inflamed, sensitive gums
- Mouth ulcers
- Cracks at the corners of the lips
- Irritation of throat and tonsils that leads to recurring infections

TEETH

- Sensitive to hot, cold, or acidic foods
- Dental cavities
- Tendency to crack or chip
- Pain in the nerves of the teeth
- Acids attack teeth externally (through acidic foods and saliva) and internally (acidic blood)

STOMACH

- Excess stomach acid
- Acid regurgitation
- Stomach pains and spasms
- Gastritis
- Ulcers

INTESTINES

- Diarrhea attacks that expel acids
- Rectal burning sensation
- Predisposition to intestinal inflammation (enteritis, colitis)
- Discoloration of the stools from liver exhaustion
- Anal fistula and cracking
- Tendency to diarrhea
- Cramps and abdominal pains

KIDNEYS AND BLADDER

- Acidic urine
- Burning and irritation in the bladder or urethra

- Excessive urination due to renal irritation
- Kidney and bladder stones

RESPIRATORY SYSTEM

- Runny nose
- Extreme sensitivity of respiratory tract to cold
- Prone to chills
- Frequent colds and bronchitis
- Sinusitis
- Angina (chest pain)
- Laryngitis
- Enlarged tonsils
- Adenoids
- Allergic tendencies
- Coughs and sore throats caused by irritation

SKIN

- Acidic sweat
- Dry skin
- Skin tends to be red and irritated in regions where there are heavy concentrations of sweat (knees, elbows, underarms, around the waist, under the band of a wristwatch or under rings that tarnish) or around openings (eyes, mouth, anus, vulva)
- Skin splits and cracks between fingers and at fingernails
- Fungal diseases
- Hives
- Itches
- Pimples
- Variety of types of eczema, but most commonly dry eczema

NAILS AND HAIR

- Nails are thin and split and break easily
- White streaks or spots on nails
- Hair looks dull, has split ends, and falls out in noticeable quantities

MUSCLES

- Leg cramps and spasms
- Stiff neck and a general sensation of aching all over
- Muscles at the nape of the neck and shoulders tend to be hard and painful

SKELETAL AND JOINT SYSTEM

- Mineral and calcium depletion of the skeleton
- Osteoporosis
- Rickets
- Tendency toward fractures (hip bone), which are slow to heal
- Joints crack
- Joint hyperlaxity
- Locking vertebrae
- Rheumatism
- Arthritis
- Sciatica
- Slipped vertebrae
- Herniated disks
- Inflammation and hardening of the ligaments
- Tendinitis
- Migrant joint pains
- Lumbar pains
- Gout

CIRCULATORY SYSTEM

- Low blood pressure
- Poor circulation
- Tendency to feel cold
- Tendency to suffer from anemia and internal bleeding
- Chilblains
- Rapid heartbeat

ENDOCRINE GLANDS

31

- Exhaustion and poor function of glands generally, except for the thyroid, which tends to be overactive

GENITAL ORGANS

- Inflammation of the genital tract by acids and infections (itching, swelling, inflammation of the uterus or vulva)
- Vaginal discharge

NERVOUS SYSTEM

- Acute sensitivity to pain anywhere in the body
- Tenacious or migrant nerve pain
- Insomnia
- Nevritis (tennis elbow)

TEST 3: FOOD ANALYSIS

Acids do not appear spontaneously in the organism but have a very specific source: they come from food intake—everything we eat, drink, and swallow (including medications and drugs).

Acids are already contained in some foods, such as rhubarb and lemons. Other acids form only when a food is being metabolized as a result of the breakdown of proteins (uric and phosphoric acids), fats (fatty acids, acetylacetic acids), carbohydrates (pyruvic and succinic acids), and so forth.

An analysis of your regular diet determines the proportion of acidifying to alkalizing foods. If your intake of alkaline elements is higher than your intake of acids, there is no risk to the body of losing its acid–alkaline balance. To the contrary, it will be greatly supported in its efforts to maintain this balance, thanks to the excess alkaline elements.

When your acid intake is higher than that of your alkaline intake, however, your acid–alkaline equilibrium is dangerously compromised, and the body receives little of the assistance it needs to restore balance from the foods it consumes. It is then obliged to find a balance using its own regulatory systems— in other words, by oxidizing, transporting, and eliminating excess acids.

The food analysis test is useful to verify whether the quantity of acidifying foods you're eating is higher or lower than that of alkaline foods. To do this, you need to establish a standard menu with variations that represent your daily diet.

To do a food analysis, keep a food diary, noting everything you consume in the course of a twenty-four-hour period. Be sure to include beverages and such incidentals as bread and between-meal snacks. Over the course of a few weeks you should notice patterns in your eating that could likely be described as two or three main menus.

In the sample menus provided below, the time of the meal is arbitrary; it serves only to distinguish between the various meals of the day. The variations possible during a particular meal are separated by the word "or." There is no need to get lost in the details. For example, it is sufficient to note "cooked vegetables" or "raw vegetables," because (unless it is tomatoes), whether these vegetables are cabbage or carrots, they are alkaline foods, and that is what concerns us here. On the other hand, "beverage" or "dessert" is too imprecise, because a beverage or dessert is either acidifying or alkalizing depending on its composition. Likewise, there is no need to make a distinction between beef, pork, and chicken, but it is important to note whether the protein source for a meal is meat or cheese or eggs. Also, you don't need to measure quantities precisely; approximations are fine.

To indicate which foods belong to which group, in the example below acidifying foods are in *italic type*, alkalizing foods are in normal type, and weak-acid foods are in bold type. Lists of these three different kinds of foods can be found on pages 52, 57, and 60, respectively.

EXAMPLES OF STANDARD MEALS

6:30 AM EITHER 1 large glass of water with **lemon**
         OR   *black coffee*

7:00 AM EITHER *whole grain bread (3 slices)* + butter + *jelly* +
                 2 coffees + milk + *2 teaspoons sugar per cup*

         OR   *cereal flakes* + milk + piece of **fresh fruit** +
                 mint tea with no sugar

         OR   **plain yogurt** + orange juice

9:00 AM EITHER apple
         OR   *coffee + croissant*
         OR   *half a chocolate bar*
         OR   almonds + raisins

Beverage: EITHER 1 quart of water in the morning
           OR   *2 or 3 coffees + cream + sugar*

33

Noon	EITHER	*meat dish + grain dish + vegetable + custard + coffee + cream + sugar*
	OR	*ham sandwich + glass of soda*
	OR	*cereal + cooked vegetables + salad*
	OR	*fish + potatoes + raw vegetables + **fresh fruit***
Beverage		water OR wine OR *lemonade* OR soda
	OR	herb tea without sugar
4:00 PM	EITHER	*bread + chocolate (pain au chocolat)*
	OR	*pastry + coffee*
	OR	*cracker + tea + teaspoon sugar*
	OR	*lemonade*
	OR	**fresh fruit**
	OR	dried fruits + water
7:00 PM	EITHER	*two-egg omelet + brown bread + green salad*
	OR	homemade vegetable soup + *crackers* + *Swiss cheese*
	OR	*cold cuts + white bread + wine*
	AND/OR	*fruit tart + whipped cream + coffee + cream + sugar*
9:00 PM	EITHER	*peanuts* OR almonds OR *crackers*
	OR	*glass of milk*
	OR	**plain yogurt**

Once you've established your standard menu, the kinds of foods that predominate in your diet will be clear. If you have difficulty metabolizing acids, you should determine whether weak-acid foods and acidifying foods outweigh alkaline foods. Otherwise you simply need to see whether your intake of acidifying foods is higher than your intake of alkalizing and weak-acid foods (these latter two have an alkalizing effect on people with no metabolic problems with acids). Detailed analyses of standard menus are provided in chapter 5.

TEST 4: LIFESTYLE ANALYSIS

In addition to diet, the manner in which you live your daily life has an influence on your acid–alkaline balance. A lifestyle analysis test is not sufficient on its own, however, to determine whether your internal environment is acidified. It should be used only as a complement to the other tests.

Because it is difficult to determine with any certainty at what point a behavior or activity stops being beneficial and becomes acidifying, the chart below describes extremes of behavior.

ACIDIFYING VS. ALKALIZING LIFESTYLES

Acidifying	Alkalizing (maintaining acid–alkaline balance)
sedentary lifestyle	active lifestyle
takes the elevator	walks up the stairs
travels mostly by car	travels on foot as much as possible
passive hobbies	active leisure-time pursuits
spends most of the time indoors	spends much time outdoors
stressed	calm, takes his or her time
restless, always short on time	relaxed and organized
sleep-deprived	gets plenty of sleep
restless sleep, insomnia	sleeps soundly
smokes	does not smoke
pessimistic	optimistic
loses temper easily, irritable	serene, patient
aggressive, envious, jealous	confident, tranquil

TEST 5: EXPERIMENTAL VERIFICATION

If acidification of the body prompts the appearance of many physical and mental problems, deacidifying the internal environment should logically bring about their disappearance. Of course, such change takes place gradually, beginning with the recent, more superficial problems and continuing with more serious, deep-rooted conditions that are caused by lesions.

Rapidly removing superficial acid from the body—the procedure explained here—will enable you to verify whether the problems you are experiencing are due to acidification of the internal environment. If the easily reversed conditions—such as nervous irritation, chronic fatigue, skin inflammation, red blotches, heartburn and similar sensations, itching, and so forth—diminish significantly or totally disappear after five to ten days of deacidification, then you can safely assume they were caused by acids. On the other hand, if this alkalization treatment does not bring about a noticeable improvement in your well-being, the problems are in all likelihood caused by something other than acidification of the internal environment.

Rapid, superficial deacidification can be achieved through a massive intake of alkaline minerals in the very easily assimilated form of alkaline citrates. The specified daily dosage of these alkaline supplements should bring an acid pH of 5 or 6 back to the normal value of 7 to 7.5.

The complete procedure is explained in detail in chapter 7. Briefly, you begin the test by taking a half-teaspoonful of powdered alkaline citrate concentrate three times a day, or three tablets before each meal with water, then gradually increase the dosage until your urinary pH has returned to 7 or 7.5. Once you have determined this ideal dosage, you should maintain it for the five to ten days. Taking a larger amount of alkaline citrates, so the urinary pH rises above 7.5, would be useless because the body cannot utilize the excess. It will simply flush the alkalines out in the urine without benefiting from them.

If your urinary pH is higher than 7 you should also perform this test, because, as explained earlier, a urinary pH with a reading higher than 7 does not necessarily mean that the internal environment of the body is not acid. The dosage of alkaline citrates should be set at two teaspoonfuls of powder three times a day or six tablets three times a day.

Rapid improvement of the problems from which you have been suffering means your body is ill because of a lack of alkaline elements, which is making your body's internal environment acid.

TEST 6: DETECTING INABILITY TO METABOLIZE ACIDS

This test is specifically indicated to determine whether you have a metabolic inability to handle acids. It is based on the same principles as the previous test, but instead of taking alkaline supplements you temporarily increase your intake of acid foods—not *acidifying* foods, but weak-acid foods such as fruits, vinegar, and whey. The acids from these foods are the most poorly metabolized by people suffering from this deficiency, so increasing intake of these acids will cause such people to experience temporary discomfort.

The purpose of this "challenge" test is not to make you sick, but simply to confirm or rule out the possibility that you have a deficiency in metabolizing acids. If you do, a more significant intake of acids should cause joint pains to intensify, red blotches on the skin to grow larger, fatigue to become more noticeable, and nervousness, burning urination, itching, and other symptoms to increase.

This test involves consuming generous helpings of fresh fruit, fruit juices, yogurts, whey products, and so forth for one or two days. This is long enough to bring about noticeable aggravation of symptoms. If you are extremely sensitive, the negative effects of acids may manifest as quickly as a half-hour to an hour after consumption. You will experience a general sense of feeling unwell and a sudden onset of fatigue, and your teeth may feel on edge in response to the aggressive acids.

Fortunately, it is not often necessary to perform this test. It is usually enough to recall what happened in the past under similar circumstances. For example, you may have seen negative effects after you ate a large quantity of fruit when it was in season, or a significant quantity of vinegar or yogurt. If you underwent a grape or lemon juice fast in the past, did it have a beneficial effect on your general health, restore your strength, and bring about the disappearance of illnesses? Or did it accentuate your symptoms and reduce your vitality?

In the first instance there is no case for a metabolic deficiency regarding acids, and it is clear that the primary causes for your state of acidification are acidifying foods and lifestyle choices. You can therefore eat weak-acid foods, for they will have an alkalizing effect.

In the second instance, though, it would be clear that you have a metabolic weakness. You can assess the degree of the problem by the intensity of the aggravation of your symptoms. You should keep close watch not only over the quantity of acidifying foods in your diet, but also the amount of weak-acid foods you consume.

Part Two

DIMINISHING ACIDIFICATION THROUGH DIET

3

Acidifying, Alkalizing, and Weak-Acid Foods

Diet is the principal source of the acid and alkaline substances that determine the acid–alkaline balance or imbalance of the body. It is therefore indispensable to have full knowledge of the properties of the foods you eat and to know precisely whether a given food has an alkalizing or acidifying effect on you personally.

In these next chapters, which are devoted to diet, the study of foods is presented in three stages.

This chapter begins with the three main groups into which food can be divided: acidifying foods, alkalizing foods, and weak-acid foods. This is not the most common division—as a rule only the first two groups are distinguished—but, as explained previously, individuals with a metabolic inability to handle acids need to be able to distinguish *acidifying* from *weak-acid* foods.

The acidifying or alkalizing nature of foods can vary enormously within one food category—for example, between different fruits and grains. Chapter 4 takes a more intensive look at these differences, tackling each kind of food and drink in turn and defining its strong, average, or weak acidifying qualities more precisely, so you can make a more judicious selection of foods when establishing your daily menus.

Chapter 5 examines menus for different meals, starting with a look at which menus for these meals—breakfast, snack, lunch, afternoon snack, and dinner—are now most common, and exploring their generally acidifying nature. This is followed by sample alkaline menus for good meals that will help restore the ideal acid–alkaline balance.

All the foods we eat can be divided into three basic groups: acidifying foods, alkalizing foods, and weak-acid foods. The definitions of the first two groups are based on the effects these foods have on the body—either acidifying or alkalizing—whereas the criterion for the third group is based on a fundamental characteristic of the food—its high content of weak acids—and does not consider its effect on the body. What is the reason for this difference?

As much as possible the characteristics of foods should always be defined based on their effects on the body rather than their intrinsic qualities, as it is the effects that people who are concerned about their health need to know. In fact, a food can display alkaline characteristics yet have an acidifying effect on the body. This is the case with white sugar, which is used to moderate the acid in the highly acidic tastes of certain fruits such as rhubarb or black currant. While this neutralization is very real on the level of taste, it vanishes when it comes to the body. When metabolized, white sugar produces numerous acids and is therefore strongly acidifying. In matters of therapeutic treatment it is very important to recognize the decisive nature of this effect.

A great mistake made by some dietitians is to consider only chemical analyses of foods and to assume that the body greatly benefits from the nutritive qualities revealed by these analyses.

The great French nutritionist and naturopath P. V. Marchesseau once said, "Food has no intrinsic value. The only value it possesses comes from the digestive tract that receives it." How should we define the quality of a food such as grass, for example, when it is good or bad depending on whether it enters the digestive tract of a cow or a human being? The same holds true for foods appropriate for people: raw vegetables are good for someone in good health, but not for a patient with enteritis or colitis. For the latter, the coarse nature of the vegetable fiber causes even greater irritation to an already-inflamed digestive tract. Dairy products are beneficial for most people, but not for those who are lactose intolerant, and so forth.

Knowing the effects a food has on the body is of fundamental importance. The foods in the first two groups, acidifying and alkalizing, have been classified according to their observed effects on human beings.

The effect of foods in the third group, that of weak-acid foods, cannot be clearly defined, unlike that of the first two groups. It varies according to the individual body's ability to metabolize acids. These foods, primarily fruits, whey, and vinegar, have an alkalizing effect on those whose bodies properly metabolize weak acids, but are acidifying for those whose bodies metabolize acids poorly, if at all. As these foods cannot be classified according to their effects, they are defined by the intrinsic characteristic of their acids, which are weak acids.

Generally speaking, the foods from this group are associated with foods that have alkalizing qualities, because that is their effect on the majority of people who eat them. But it would be a serious error to adopt that as the sole classification, because, on the one hand, it does not entirely correspond to the reality, and on the other, most people who are concerned about their acid–alkaline balance have a metabolic weakness toward acids. For them, knowledge of this third group is crucial.

Understanding these three groups permits you to select without risk of error the foods that are necessary to add to your diet to restore the ideal acid–alkaline balance. You should choose foods according to these two rules of thumb:

- If your body metabolizes acids properly, the quantity of alkalizing and weak-acid foods should be higher than the quantity of acidifying foods.

- If you have a metabolic inability to handle acids, the quantity of alkalizing foods should be higher than the quantity of acidifying and weak-acid foods.

Two points need to be emphasized. First, the more a person is afflicted by acidification or a metabolic inability to handle acids, the higher should be the proportion of alkalizing foods in the diet in proportion to the others. In fact, while a person with a healthy acid–alkaline balance can eat acidifying and alkaline foods in equal amounts, people with an imbalance should make alkalizing foods 60 to 80 percent of their diet.

Reducing acidifying foods drastically or eliminating them completely would not be wise, because foods rich in proteins (eggs, dairy products, meat, fish) are among the acidifying group. An adequate intake of proteins is a prerequisite for alkaline minerals to establish themselves properly in the tissues. Tissues require proteins to produce a good framework to contain the minerals. Otherwise, a portion of the alkaline minerals ingested will leave the body and will therefore be unavailable when the body needs them to neutralize acids.

Second, the more you suffer from problems caused by acidification or a metabolic inability to handle acids, the greater the necessity to consume a more significant amount of alkaline foods *at every meal.* If you include those foods in every meal of the day, neutralization of food acids or acids produced in the digestive process is handled directly by the alkaline elements contributed by the food just eaten.

This intake represents a valuable aid to the body, for without it food acids leave the intestinal tract and enter the internal environment, forcing the body to draw from its tissue reserves the alkaline elements it requires to neutralize them. This results in a depletion of the body's mineral content and prompts the appearance of health conditions caused by acidification.

People who can metabolize acids properly are less subject to the necessity of eating more alkaline foods than acid foods. They have good reserves of alkaline elements that can be drawn on when needed to neutralize the acids from a meal that consists exclusively or almost exclusively of acidifying foods.

ACIDIFYING FOODS

Acidifying foods are primarily those that are rich in proteins, carbohydrates, fats, or some combination of the three.

ACIDIFYING FOODS

- Meat, poultry, cold cuts, meat extracts, fish, seafood (mussels, shrimp)
- Eggs

- Cheeses (strong cheeses are more acidic than mild cheeses)
- Animal fats such as lard and suet
- Vegetable oils, especially peanut oil and oils that are refined or hardened (margarine)
- Whole grains and refined grains: wheat, oats, especially millet
- Bread, pasta, cereal flakes, and foods with a grain base
- Leguminous plants such as peanuts, soybeans, white beans, broad beans
- White sugar
- Sweets: syrups, pastry, chocolate, candy, jelly, fruit preserves
- Oleaginous fruits: walnuts, hazelnuts, pumpkin seeds
- Commercially manufactured sweet drinks, primarily sodas
- Coffee, tea, cocoa, wine
- Condiments such as mayonnaise, mustard, and ketchup

Foods rich in proteins (meat, dairy products, and leguminous plants) are acidifying because their digestion produces amino acids; and because proteins, once they have been utilized by the body's cells, engender products of acidic degradation. Uric acid, for example, primarily comes from the proteins that serve in the construction of the cell core and are found in foods consisting of cells, such as animal meats. Unlike meat and fish, dairy products do not carry uric acid because milk and cheese are not composed of animal tissues. Furthermore, the essential amino acids that make up animal meats always contain phosphorus and sulfur, two acid minerals.

Although they are not composed of animal tissue, the leguminous plants (soybeans, chickpeas) bring a large quantity of uric acid into the body because they are rich in purines. Intrinsically alkaline, these purines are transformed into uric acid so they may be eliminated from the body. The presence of large amounts of purines in coffee, tea, and cocoa also explains why these beverages, as well as chocolate, are acidifying.

The acidifying nature of foods rich in fats (animal fat used in cooking, the fat contained in meat, deep-frying oil) is twofold. First, fat is utilized by the body in the form of *fatty acids;* and secondly, *saturated* fatty acids—which animal-based foods contain in great quantity—are difficult to metabolize. When their digestion is incomplete they create toxic acid substances such as acetones, acetylacetic acid, beta-hydroxybutyric acid, and others. These waste products and metabolic residues appear only if fat breakdown in the body is faulty; normal digestion of fats yields fatty acids. As fat consumption is rather high in today's standard diet, acidification from fats is all too common.

The acidifying properties of carbohydrates are due to the same types of processes that are involved with fat and its acidic nature. In the form of starch,

42

carbohydrates are actually aggregates of thousands of glucose molecules—up to 250,000 of them—whereas it takes only several hundred amino acids to produce a protein. For the body to use carbohydrates they must be broken down into increasingly smaller fragments until they are reduced to their basic constituent element: the glucose molecule.

The greatest culprit in the production of acids is the poor conversion of long chains of glucose. Just like fat and proteins, carbohydrates go through various stages of transformation during which their characteristic properties change what was originally alkaline into an acid. If these conversions are interrupted while in progress the body becomes acidified, because the intermediary acid substances are not converted back into alkaline substances, as would be the normal end result of this process. This breakdown of the process is all too common, since the overconsumption of carbohydrates (bread, cereals, pastas, crackers) is quite significant and often goes well beyond the body's capacity to digest them properly. The problem is the same whether the process involves whole grains or refined grains.

While cereal grains are acidifying, germinated grains are not. In fact, because of the radical transformation of their composition due to the germination process, these foods are considered to be alkalizing and are classified with green vegetables, since young grain sprouts are more or less green when eaten. This is also the case for the sprouts of leguminous plants such as soybeans, lentils, and chickpeas. (Bread made with sprouted grains, however, is not alkalizing.)

White sugar, a carbohydrate that consists of only two molecules (glucose and fructose), is acidifying for a different reason. Its acidifying nature, and that of the foods containing it (jellies, candies, chocolate, cookies), comes from the fact that it is refined and stripped of all trace elements, vitamins, and enzymes; it is thus generally poorly converted by the body. The body cannot indefinitely continue releasing large quantities of vitamins and trace elements to produce the conversion of sugar into energy. The average annual consumption of white sugar today is more than ninety pounds per person, which is more than the body can handle. The transformation of sugar in the body inevitably stalls at one of the intermediary acidic stages.

Refined white sugar and all the products that contain it are strongly acidifying, but the naturally occurring sugars of fruits and vegetables (like carrots and beets) are not. This is because the tissues of fruits and vegetables contain all the necessary trace elements, vitamins, and enzymes necessary to complete their transformation in the body. For the same reasons, whole sugar, meaning the concentrate obtained from the evaporation of sugar-cane sap, is not acidifying either. Brown sugars, on the other hand, have undergone several refining processes that have depleted their vitamin and trace element content. Consequently, they too are acidifying, and the closer they are to white sugar (the most acidic form of sugar), the more acidifying their effect is on the body. The fructose or fruit sugar available for sale commercially is also depleted of all its naturally occurring vitamin content, making it an acidifying agent as well.

Oleaginous fruits (except for almonds and Brazil nuts) are all acidifying, including walnuts, hazelnuts, cashews, pecans, coconut, and even the seeds used in health food mixes—sunflower seeds, pumpkin seeds, sesame seeds, and so forth. Their acidifying character is due to their high fat content as well as their high content of protein, phosphorus, and sulfur. However, a few sunflower seeds do not acidify the body to the same extent as six to twelve ounces of meat, although both foods are included in the list of acidifying foods.

Based on their characteristics, the foods in the acidifying group have an acidifying effect on everyone who eats them, unlike weak-acid foods, which may have an acidifying or alkalizing effect depending on the individual's physical capabilities. The manner in which the body utilizes acidifying foods inevitably leads to the production of acids, so it is advisable to pay strict attention to the amount of acidifying foods you include in your daily diet if you want to avoid acidification of your internal environment. This does not mean a complete elimination of these items from the diet, or even an extreme reduction. It is simply a matter of keeping the quantity of acidifying foods lower than that of alkalizing foods. This should be a general guideline for what you eat every day or, even better, for what you eat at every meal.

ALKALIZING FOODS

Alkalizing foods consist primarily of green and colored vegetables (with the exception of tomatoes) and potatoes.

These foods are alkalizing because they are rich in alkaline elements and contain few, if any, acid substances, and because they do not produce acids when they are utilized by the body. Even when significant amounts of this type of food are consumed, no acid is produced, regardless of the metabolic capacities of the person who eats them. Just as acidifying foods are acidifying for everyone, alkalizing foods are alkalizing for everyone. These are the foods that people suffering from an acid–alkaline imbalance need to eat above all.

Green and colored vegetables are the primary source of alkaline substances for the body. They should be included in every main meal, whether as salad, raw or cooked vegetables, juice, or soup, by anyone trying to restore or maintain acid–alkaline balance. The sole exception is the tomato, which is very acidifying whether eaten raw or cooked. (Botanically speaking, however, the tomato is not a vegetable but a fruit.)

ALKALIZING FOODS

- Potatoes
- Green vegetables, raw or cooked: salad greens, green beans, cabbage, and so on
- Colored vegetables: carrots, beets (except for tomatoes)

44

- Corn (kernels or cooked as polenta)
- Milk (liquid and powdered form), large-curd cottage cheese, cream, butter
- Bananas
- Almonds, Brazil nuts
- Chestnuts
- Dried fruits: dates, raisins (except for those that are acidic to the taste—apricots, apples, pineapple)
- Alkaline mineral waters
- Almond milk
- Black olives preserved in oil
- Avocado
- Cold-pressed oils
- Natural sugar

Potatoes are well known for their anti-acidifying qualities; their juice is often recommended as a remedy for stomach acidity and ulcers. The potato's wealth of alkaline elements makes it the best choice of foods to counter the acidification of the body. A starchy food, it is nourishing and a beneficial alternative to cereal grains, which are acidifying. A deacidifying diet must include potatoes more often than foods from cereal grains.

Another nourishing and valuable food for fighting excess acidity is the chestnut. Like the potato, it is starchy, it supplies fuel for energy, and it is not acidifying like cereal grains. Chestnuts can be roasted in the oven or boiled in water and eaten as a vegetable. The best-known recipe containing them is probably red cabbage with chestnuts. Like potatoes, chestnuts go well with cheese. But watch out for chestnut purees, which are often sweetened with sugar.

Of all the fruits, the banana is the only one that is truly alkalizing, because its own acid content is so weak that it never causes acidification, even when consumed in large quantities or as a regular part of the diet. Other fruits, in contrast, even those that are only faintly acid, such as melons, do contain acids, which means that the more one eats of them, the greater the acidifying effect they have.

Generally speaking, dried fruits (dates, raisins) are alkalizing because a portion of their acid content is oxidized in the drying process. They are less alkalizing if they are set out to dry before reaching full maturity, as is often the case with apples and apricots. The alkaline nature of dried fruits is also slightly reduced when they are treated with sulfur as a preservative.

Almonds and Brazil nuts are the only alkalizing oleaginous fruits. They can be eaten just as they are, or chopped or sliced and mixed with salads, vegetables, and desserts. Some dietetic and health food stores sell a sugarless almond paste, which can be mixed with water to make almond milk, a very pleasant and alkalizing beverage.

Black olives preserved in olive oil are alkalizing, unlike those, either black or green, that are preserved in a vinegar-based brine.

Raw or whole sugar is not alkalizing, properly speaking, meaning that it does not alkalize the internal environment if eaten in large quantities, but when eaten in moderation it does not acidify either, as is the case with other sugars. Likewise, corn, milk, large-curd cottage cheese, cream, butter, and so on, eaten in moderation, do not acidify the body.

Water usually has a pH of 7. Carbonated mineral water is acid, because the gas that gives it its carbonation is carbonic acid. The principal alkaline mineral waters—those with a pH above 7—are Limpia Water (Italy), Contrexéville and Évian (France), and Henniez bleue (Switzerland). To determine whether a mineral water is alkaline, read the label on the bottle, as the pH is indicated there.

WEAK-ACID FOODS

This group consists of foods whose alkalizing or acidifying effect depends on the metabolic capacities of the person who eats them. Their classification is therefore not based upon their physical effect (because that cannot be defined in advance) but on the basic nature of their acids, which are weak acids.

These foods contain a good deal of acid, hence their acidic taste. Because the acids in them are weak, for people capable of metabolizing them properly by easily oxidizing them, they are transformed into alkaline elements and therefore contribute to the alkalization of the body. But for people whose metabolisms cannot handle acids properly, the large quantity of acids contained in these foods is not oxidized, and they thus will have an acidifying effect.

The primary weak-acid foods are fruits, whey, and vinegar.

WEAK-ACID FOODS

- Whey, yogurt, curds, kefir, small-curd cottage cheese
- Unripe fruits (the less ripe a fruit, the higher its acid content)
- Acid fruits: berries (red and black currants, raspberries, strawberries); citrus fruits (lemons, grapefruit, tangerines, oranges); certain varieties of apples (Winesap), cherries (Morello), plums, apricots
- Sweet fruits (especially when eaten in excess), melon, watermelon
- Acid vegetables: tomato, rhubarb, sorrel, watercress
- Sauerkraut, vegetables that have been lactofermented (cultured with *Lactobacillus*)

- Fruit juices, lemon juice (in salad dressing)
- Honey
- Vinegar

The faintly acid taste of apples and pears, or the strongly acidic flavor of lemons and red currants, is indicative of how high or low their acid content is. For these foods the sense of taste can be used to determine the degree of acidity. The acid content is higher in unripe fruit: the less ripe it is, the more acid. Fruits that are perfectly ripe have the least acidity. Apricots, for example, are extremely acid before maturity, even if their color is already orange, but are alkaline when they become ripe and mellow. Even within a single species of fruit, for example apples or cherries, the degree of acidity of the fruit varies according to the variety; Winesap apples are more acidic than Golden Delicious apples, Morello cherries are more acidic than Bing cherries, and so forth.

Drinking fruit juice as an alternative to eating the flesh of the fruit does not reduce the acid—on the contrary. Alkaline minerals are primarily located in the pulp and remain there when the fruits are squeezed for juice. Since they are not present in the juice, they cannot neutralize its acidity. (This is not the case for juices made with an electric [centrifuge] juicer, as they contain pulverized pulp.) The consumption of fruits in the form of juice can also distort your impression of how much fruit you are eating. You probably do not eat more than two oranges at one sitting, but you can easily drink two or three glasses of orange juice at a time, the equivalent of six to eight oranges.

Cooking fruits also does not diminish their acidity. In the majority of cases, cooking simply increases the acidity because the heat destroys some of the vitamins and enzymes. Furthermore, most cooked fruit dishes have white sugar added, and we have already discussed the highly acidic properties of that food.

The case of whey is unique. This food, which consists of the liquid part of milk that has been curdled through fermentation, is a transparent, clear yellow liquid. It is found in fresh white cheeses like cottage or farmer cheese, yogurt (whey is the liquid that collects in the impression made by a spoon in yogurt), kefir, and so on. When fresh, whey is alkaline, but after an hour or two it becomes acid. It primarily creates lactic acid, which, like the acids found in fruits, is relatively easy for the body to oxidize and convert into an alkaline substance, so long as the individual has no trouble metabolizing acids. When there is a metabolic inability to handle acids, however, the acids are not converted and therefore contribute to the acidification of the body's internal environment. People with this metabolic deficiency have to monitor their intake of whey, yogurt, and kefir just as they do that of fruits.

The acid fermentation used to make yogurt can also be used to preserve vegetables or juices. Sauerkraut, lactofermented vegetables and vegetable juices, and vinegar, for the same reasons that apply to the foods we have just discussed, are acidifying for those with metabolism difficulties with acids but are alkalizing for everyone else.

Honey is moderately acidic.

The acidifying or alkalizing nature of fruits, whey, and vinegar is the subject of constant debate. Of course, people whose metabolisms have no problem with acids are convinced of the alkalizing nature of these foods, while the rest remain equally convinced of their acidifying nature based on their personal experience. There is no reason for this controversy ever to have arisen. These foods can be either acidifying or alkalizing, and as such they form this distinct third group of weak-acid foods.

In cases of extreme acidification, there is no need to worry that the total removal of all fruits from the diet will result in an insufficient intake of vitamins, as some have claimed. Fruit is certainly an extraordinary source of vitamins, but vegetables contain many as well—quite a broad spectrum, in fact. Because vegetables are the foundation of the diet of those suffering from acidification, the amount they consume should cover their daily vitamin requirements.

In fact, the elimination of weak-acid foods will not cause major problems, because none of them is absolutely indispensable, unlike some foods with acidifying properties. Fresh fruits can be replaced with dried fruits, dairy products rich in whey by those containing none, and lactofermented vegetables by fresh vegetables. In practice, it is often necessary for a person suffering from this kind of metabolism deficiency to completely eliminate weak-acid foods from the diet for several weeks to a month. This restriction has never created problems (other than the person's yearning to eat a food from this group that she or he enjoys). But the benefits of the deacidification more than compensate for the temporary sacrifice.

EIGHT RULES FOR AN ACID–ALKALINE BALANCED DIET

There are four elementary principles for selecting foods to ensure a proper balance of acidifying, alkalizing, and weak-acid foods. The four additional rules are for those who are unable to metabolize acids properly.

- Rule one: A meal should never consist solely of acidifying foods but should always contain alkaline foods.

A meal of meat with pasta, or fish and rice, with cake and coffee for dessert is not a recommended menu because it consists entirely of acidifying foods; the same applies to a meatless meal of pasta with tomato sauce followed by a dessert sweetened with white sugar. When vegetables are added to this meal in the form of salads or raw or cooked vegetables, the alkaline intake at least partially compensates for the acids. Vegetables are typically included with meals, but often in such small quantities that their effect is negligible. This takes us to rule number two.

48

- Rule two: The amount of alkalizing foods should be greater proportionately than the amount of acidifying foods at any one meal.

The proportion of foods that produce alkaline elements should always be greater than that of foods that produce acids. Eating in this manner ensures that the acids are neutralized at the intestinal or tissue level without any need for the body to draw from its reserves.

- Rule three: The proportion of alkalizing foods should be even greater when there is pronounced acidification of the internal environment or when the individual is unable to metabolize acids properly.

The more the body is weakened or exhausted, the less the alkaline reserves it has for its buffer system, and the less capable it is of oxidizing acids. Putting less acid into the body makes it easier for the body to maintain its acid–alkaline balance.

- Rule four: A diet consisting solely of alkaline vegetables and plant-based food is possible, but only for a limited period (one to two weeks).

An exclusively alkaline diet, consisting solely of vegetables, potatoes, bananas, almonds, and so forth, cannot be continued indefinitely because it is seriously inadequate in protein. Such diets are useful when acidification is very significant and the disorders it has caused are acute, intense, and painful. The abrupt, complete elimination of all acids allows the body to recover more rapidly and return to a normal acid–alkaline balance. An exclusively alkaline diet should remain a short-term therapeutic action so as not to compromise health.

There are four additional rules that people suffering from an inability to metabolize weak acids properly should heed.

- Rule five: A meal should never consist solely of acid foods but should always include alkaline foods.

This rule is almost identical to rule one, but it involves weak-acid foods rather than acidifying foods. Eating fruits and yogurt exclusively or drinking only whey-based beverages is strongly discouraged, as the acid intake from such a diet is not compensated by any alkaline food, and the body must draw these substances from its own tissues. The risk of health problems caused by mineral depletion is therefore quite significant. These manifest as a sudden drop in vitality, the feeling that one's teeth are on edge, a chilly sensation, itching, joint pains, and other symptoms that have been discussed previously.

Alkaline foods that are good accompaniments to fresh fruits are fresh (unripened) cheeses, soft white cheese (large-curd cottage cheese, low-fat cream cheese, ricotta, quark, mozzarella, farmer cheese, fresh goat cheese, yogurt cheese), cream, almonds, bananas, and salad greens. Fresh fruits can also be mixed with raw vegetables.

- Rule six: The quantities of weak-acid and acidifying foods a person eats should be tailored to meet his or her personal metabolic capabilities.

The inability to metabolize weak acids properly is rarely absolute; it varies according to individual physiology as well as circumstances (such as stress, fatigue, work, and vacations). Each person has a certain rate at which he or she can metabolize acids properly at any given time, a rate that cannot be surpassed without overtaxing the body's capacity.

As long as the quantity of acids ingested or created by the digestion of food is below this rate, the body manages to neutralize them through oxidation before any of the health problems created by acidification manifest. Accordingly, for certain extremely sensitive individuals, half a Golden Delicious apple—no more—suits them just fine, but even a quarter of a Winesap apple is more than they can handle. For any given person, a certain quantity of a food can be acidifying, yet alkalizing or neutral in a lesser amount.

So if you have difficulty metabolizing acids, you can safely eat weak-acid foods as long as you tailor the amount you consume to your physical capacities. Your tolerance threshold can also change over time. You can discover and keep track of your own threshold through experimentation and observation.

- Rule seven: Weak-acid foods should not be eaten too rapidly in succession.

An individual with an inability to metabolize weak acids properly, but with a normal acid–alkaline balance, can generally handle a sudden increase in weak-acid intake (from eating a large quantity of fruit, for example) by drawing from the body's reserves, provided that this kind of event is the exception and not the rule. In fact, if the withdrawal of alkaline substances from the body's reserves is a unique event, the acid–alkaline balance is not endangered, and no acidification problem will occur.

But some time will have to go by before the body's reserves are replenished. If eating another piece of fruit puts additional acids into the body too soon, it has to draw from its already-diminished reserves, which may not contain enough alkaline substances to neutralize the acid from the fruit; thus, acid–alkaline balance is compromised. Health problems due to acidification will appear not because the body is not intrinsically capable of neutralizing this fruit's acid—it has successfully done so before—but because the fruit has been eaten too soon after the first fruit was consumed.

By spacing out the ingestion of these hard-to-metabolize foods, you can increase your personal level of tolerance for them. This is useful to know, as it allows you to expand the selection of foods you can safely eat.

- Rule eight: Weak-acid foods must be eaten when the body is ready to receive them.

There is an Arabic proverb that says: "Oranges are like gold in the morning, silver at noon, and lead in the evening." For people with an inability to metabolize weak acids properly, the opposite is true. Oranges and fruits in general are harmful in the morning and much more beneficial at noon or in the evening. The reason for this is that by noon the body's "organic motor" has had time to warm up and is turning over naturally. In fact, some people take a long time *physically* to wake up in the morning. The heart beats more slowly, blood pressure is low, and cellular exchanges—including oxidation—take place in slow motion. The body reaches cruising speed only after several hours of activity and a meal or two. If such a person eats fruits or drinks a glass of orange juice in the morning, not only will he or she have difficulty metabolizing the acids but, because the body is still working below its real capacity, it will have even greater trouble oxidizing weak acids than it normally would.

Along the same lines of reasoning, weak-acids foods are metabolized better in the summer, when the weather is hot and sunny, as well as when one is rested (as opposed to feeling tired).

4

Classifying the Acidification Potential of Foods

In the previous chapter we divided food into three basic categories. Even within a single category, however, not all foods are uniformly alkalizing or acidifying. For example, both rice and millet are acidifying foods, but millet is much more acidifying than rice. To fine-tune an optimal diet, we need to refine these classifications.

The classification used here presents foods in a three-column chart. Vegetables are presented as very alkaline, slightly alkaline, and acidifying. Other foods are categorized as alkalizing, slightly acidifying, and very acidifying. This division helps people suffering from acidification to avoid or limit acidifying foods and to choose more strongly alkalizing foods, which are of the greatest benefit in correcting the imbalance of their internal environment.

This is not a precise hierarchical organization, where each food occupies a set place with regard to the others; we currently lack the objective criteria necessary for establishing such an exact hierarchy. Analysis of a food's chemical composition is not germane because it does not take into account what happens once the food has been ingested. As we have seen, digestion and the body's utilization of foods alter their properties. These classifications are therefore based on observation of the effects these foods have on the body.

Based on your own experience, however, you may feel one food or another is better placed in a category different than the one assigned to it here. This is not surprising, since each person's body has its own strengths and weaknesses in handling certain foods. It can in fact be the case that a food has a very acidifying effect on one person, whereas for most people its acidifying effect is weak. You are well advised to trust your own experience rather than to base all your food choices on theory.

Nonetheless, the classification on these charts is valid for the majority of people. For the rest, it can serve as a useful guide for taking the first steps while they are in the process of determining how to modify their diet according to their individual needs and the intrinsic capabilities of their own bodies.

FRESH FRUITS

The classification of fresh fruits is valid only for those who are unable to metabolize acids properly. For everyone else, all fruits have an alkalizing effect.

Because a fruit's acidifying properties depend on how ripe it is—the more ripe, the less acid—the classification assumes the fruits listed are in their ripest state. But just what is a ripe fruit, exactly?

Most people today do not have gardens or orchards, so they depend on grocery stores for their produce. But for economic reasons, most fruit sold in stores is harvested long before it reaches maturity, because fruit is less fragile (and therefore easier to ship) when still hard and green. The spoilage rate is therefore greatly reduced, and the fruit can survive the elaborate handling that takes place at the level of the producer, the wholesaler, the retail seller, and finally the consumer. Picking fruit when it is unripe also permits better management of inventory, as the flow of merchandise can easily be adapted to the needs of the market.

The harmful result of this premature harvesting is that fruit never reaches the full ripeness that makes it soft, aromatic, sweet, and juicy. If you have ever had the opportunity to taste a fruit that has ripened on the tree in the open air, bathed in the rays of the sun, you know how much more delicious it is than what you usually eat.

Aside from the question of taste, the natural ripening of fruits brings about very significant reduction in their acid content, much more than takes place in fruits harvested before they are ripe. One of my patients, who could not metabolize acids properly, loved oranges but could not eat them without experiencing discomfort. To his great surprise, when he took a trip to an orange-producing region just at the time the fruit was ripe, he found he could eat a pound or more of oranges daily without the least bit of distress. Having attained their full maturation under the sun rather than sitting in a warehouse since they were green, these oranges now contained only a very small amount of acids, which were quite easy for him to metabolize.

Every fruit is a complete entity in and of itself and should whenever possible be eaten in its entirety, skin and seeds and all. Of course, apricot kernels and cherry stones are too large to be swallowed easily and too hard to be digested. But apple, orange, and grape seeds, among others, contain elements that are of great benefit to the body and are useful to its metabolism of the fruit. Furthermore, the skin of fruits contains numerous minerals and enzymes that facilitate neutralization of the acid contained in the fruit pulp. It is thus a mistake to peel apples and pears and to get rid of the skins of figs, grapes, prunes, and so forth. Only orange and citrus fruit peel, melon rind, and pomegranate skin should be thrown away, even if they have not been treated with pesticides and other chemicals.

Fresh fruits can be eaten as they are or shredded or chopped in a fresh fruit salad. Fresh fruits are naturally sweet, so adding sugar should be avoided, because sugar is an acidifying agent. It is also best not to eat fruits along with cereal grains—for example, in granola or muesli—because the combination of fresh fruit and cereal flakes is hard to digest and encourages fermentation, which is a great producer of acid toxins.

Cooking fruit does not reduce its acidity. When cooking compotes and pies, it is important to use ripe apples and not green apples that have fallen prematurely.

Shredding or slicing fruit makes it more alkaline, because the contact of the pulp with air allows some of its acid content to oxidize.

The only alkalizing fruit, the banana, is not easily digested by everyone. This is usually because it has been picked before it has become truly ripe. A ripe banana has very sweet, soft flesh. Its sugar content can be increased by mashing it into a puree with a fork or spoon and allowing it to sit out in the air for ten to twelve minutes before eating it.

Another way to neutralize the aggressive nature of fruit-based acids is to eat them with soft white cheese, fresh cheese, or cream. This is common in many cuisines, as smaller fruits such as strawberries and raspberries are eaten with crème fraîche or sour cream.

FRESH FRUITS

Alkalizing	Slightly acidifying	Very acidifying
	FRUITS	
	Golden Delicious apples	cider, Winesap apples
	pears: Bartlett, Comice, Bosc, Seckel	other pears
	grapes	
	plums	nectarines, greengage plums
	very ripe apricots	other apricots
	Bing cherries	Morello cherries
	peaches	
	figs	
	yellow plums (mirabelles)	
	melons	
	watermelon	

BERRIES

strawberries, big and sweet	strawberries, small and tart
gooseberries	red currants in bunches
blueberries	raspberries
	black currants
	sea buckthorn
	sloe (blackthorn berries)
	mulberries

CITRUS FRUITS

clementines	mandarins
	oranges
	lemons
	citron
	grapefruit

EXOTIC FRUITS

bananas	mangos	pineapples
	pomegranates	kiwis
	persimmons	

DRIED FRUITS

Dried fruits have lost the greater portion of their water content, and thus their juice, after having been set out to dry under the sun or in an oven. Dates are an exception; they are naturally low in water, and the way they appear in the stores ready for consumption is exactly how they look when ripening on the tree.

DRIED FRUITS

Alkalizing	Slightly acidifying	Very acidifying
raisins	prunes	tart apricots, sulfur treated
sweet apricots, dried naturally	pears	
bananas	apples	
dates	peaches	
	figs	
	mangos	
	pineapple	

Because dried fruits are naturally quite sweet, they usually do not have sugar added to them before they are sold, with the exception of some dates that are packed in a sweet syrup.

Of course, the riper and sweeter a fruit is before it is dried, the higher its alkaline content after this process. The acidity of the fresh fruit is reduced in any event by the drying process, thanks to oxidation.

Dried fruits play a very small role in the average diet of most people, and many people never eat them. Because they are alkalizing, however, their consumption ought to be encouraged. They allow individuals with a high sensitivity to the acids of fresh fruits to eat fruit in a form suitable for their particular needs.

Dried fruit is extremely concentrated, and some people have trouble digesting it. Soaking the fruit in water for twelve to twenty-four hours before eating it makes it more easily digestible. It can be eaten with or without its soaking liquid.

Soaked dried fruit can also be made into delicious desserts by blending the fruit and its soaking liquid with a from-age blanc or cream cheese.

OLEAGINOUS FRUITS

As the name suggests, oleaginous fruits are rich in oil. Half their weight, in fact, consists of oil. Many people consider them to be incidental rather than staple foods and only eat them occasionally when they are part of a cake or cookie.

Of all the oleaginous fruits, only two are truly alkaline: almonds and Brazil nuts. But the alkalizing benefits of almonds are so strong that people suffering from acidification should eat them on a regular basis. Black olives are equally alkalizing, in contrast to green olives, but only if they have been preserved in oil and not in a brine or vinegar preparation.

Oleaginous fruits can be eaten just as they are, either one variety at a time or in combination, or along with dried fruits. Because of their high concentrations of basic nutrients it is better not to mix too many different kinds together, as this can make them difficult to digest. Crushed, slivered, or grated oleaginous fruits can be added to fruit salads, green salads, and raw-vegetable platters, or can be spread on bread like butter. Many different kinds of nut butters and pastes are readily available in supermarkets, groceries, and gourmet and health food stores. Peanut butter sandwiches, of course, are a lunchbox staple. Unsweetened almond paste can also be used to make almond milk. Tahini, or sesame paste, is an ingredient in many popular Middle Eastern dishes, such as hummus and baba ghanoush.

OLEAGINOUS FRUITS

Alkalizing	Slightly acidifying	Very acidifying
almonds	cashews	walnuts

56

Brazil nuts	sesame seeds	hazelnuts
black olives in oil	pine nuts	peanuts
	coconut	pecans
	green olives	pistachios
		pumpkin seeds
		sunflower seeds
		olives in brine or vinegar

VEGETABLES

Except for tomatoes and eggplants, which are quite acidifying, all vegetables are alkalizing and should make up a significant portion of your diet if you are suffering from problems caused by acidification. Some vegetables are very alkalizing, however, and others are less so. The latter have been listed in a second column under the heading "Slightly alkaline"; these are chiefly white (endive, celery, cauliflower, etc.) and sulfurous vegetables.

Sulfurous, or cruciferous, vegetables (broccoli, brussels sprouts, radishes, onions, peppers, etc.) can restore minerals to the depleted physical internal environment of a person suffering from acidification, but they also contain sulfur, which itself is acid. Among sensitive individuals the sulfur not only has a slightly acidifying effect but is also an irritant to the mucous membranes of the digestive system, as well as to the respiratory mucous membranes and the skin when the acid is eliminated—and these organs are already weakened and sensitive in people suffering from acidification. But this is of concern only if you are overly sensitive to acids, and only when you consume too large a quantity of the vegetables in question.

White and sulfurous vegetables can therefore be eaten, but to guarantee a good supply of minerals it is best to eat primarily green and colored vegetables, potatoes, and certain fruiting vegetables (cucumber, sweet pepper, etc.).

Vegetables can be eaten raw, cooked, in soup, or in juice. When you eat them raw with a dressing, be sure the dressing is not so acidic that it destroys their beneficial alkalizing qualities. Too often, such dressings contain so much vinegar or lemon juice that they not only drown out the flavor of the vegetables, but are also strongly acidifying if you are unable to metabolize acids properly. In that case you need to measure your intake of vinegar or lemon juice in teaspoons, not tablespoons. (Experiments have shown that vinegar is less acidifying than lemon juice.)

Cooked vegetables contain smaller amounts of vitamins and enzymes than raw vegetables, because cooking destroys some of that content. However, the mineral content—which is most important in terms of restoring a healthy acid–alkaline balance—is not altered when vegetables are braised, steamed, or roasted. Boiling draws minerals from the vegetables into the cooking water, which is generally thrown away after use, along with these valuable elements.

Vegetables can make up part or all of a single meal. Homemade vegetable soup is highly recommended, especially in winter, for not only does it replenish the body's mineral content (soup contains the vegetables' mineral-rich cooking liquid), but its warmth counteracts one of the most common symptoms of acidification, the feeling of always being cold (due to the depletion of minerals).

Homemade vegetable juice has more benefit than canned, since it is fresh. Commercial vegetable juices vary in freshness, depending on how they are preserved. If you have trouble metabolizing acids you should avoid juices that have been lactofermented, because they are slightly acidic.

If you make your own vegetable juice you can use a single vegetable or make a vegetable cocktail out of several different varieties. If possible, use organic produce so as to avoid ingesting chemicals. If the juice is too strong for your taste, you can dilute it with water without losing any of the alkalizing benefits. (Water has a neutral pH except when chlorinated, a process that makes it more acidic.)

VEGETABLES

Very alkaline	Slightly alkaline	Acidifying
potatoes		
GREEN VEGETABLES		
salad greens: chicory, escarole, lettuce, mâche, dandelion green cabbage celery stalks green beans fennel		

58

Very alkaline	Slightly alkaline	Acidifying
beet greens		
artichokes		
broccoli		
brussels sprouts		

COLORED VEGETABLES

Very alkaline	Slightly alkaline	Acidifying
spinach		
carrots		
red beets		
red cabbage		
yellow beans		
sweet potatoes		

FRUITING VEGETABLES

Very alkaline	Slightly alkaline	Acidifying
edible gourds	avocado	tomato
zucchini		eggplant
squash		sour pickles
cucumber		
sweet pepper		

WHITE VEGETABLES

endive
celeriac
salsify
Jerusalem artichoke
cauliflower
parsnip
Chinese artichoke

SULFUROUS VEGETABLES

radishes
turnips
peppers
onions
garlic
shallots
asparagus

CEREAL GRAINS

There are countless ways to prepare cereal grains. They can be eaten whole (rice, spelt, etc.), ground (polenta, couscous, bulgur), crushed into cereal flakes, or ground into flour to thicken sauces and soups and to make bread, biscuits, and crackers, or very finely ground to be used in cakes and pastas.

With the exception of corn, all cereals and their byproducts are acidifying. Their acidity increases in proportion to their refinement; white rice, for example, is much more acidifying than brown rice.

Of all the cereal grains, millet is the most acidifying. This is important to know, as it is often recommended for its excellent ability to replenish minerals in the case of hair loss, rheumatism, and so on because of its high silica content. However, silica is an acid mineral that is usually found in the form of silicic acid. Millet's ability to restore minerals to the body is undeniable, but people with problems digesting acid should avoid it, because its silica content is more than their bodies can deal with.

CEREAL GRAINS

Alkalizing	Slightly acidifying	Very acidifying
WHOLE GRAINS, GROUND GRAINS, GERMINATED GRAINS		
corn	wheat	millet
	brown rice	white rice
	rye	
	barley	
	spelt	
	buckwheat	
	quinoa	
	pilpil	couscous

Alkalizing	Slightly acidifying	Very acidifying
	whole semolina	semolina
	cream of rice	
BREADS		
	whole-grain bread	yeast bread
	(without yeast)	white bread
	dark bread	
CRACKERS		
	whole grain	made from white flour
PASTA		
	whole grain	made from white flour

CEREAL FLAKES	
whole-grain cereals, soaked for about 10 hours naturally baked flakes (e.g., corn flakes)	sugar frosted sweetened granola, muesli baked and sugared flakes

GRANOLA BARS	
whole grain with little sugar	with lots of sugar and/or chocolate coated

COOKIES AND CAKES	
whole grain with little sugar cake made from whole wheat	made with white flour, white sugar, chocolate pies white cake flour

White bread is more acidifying than whole-grain or dark breads because, stripped of vitamins, trace elements, and enzymes to make it more easily digestible, it produces—like white sugar—numerous acids. Yeast breads have also been included with acidifying foods, because the yeast that makes dough rise also makes it acidic, as can easily be verified by tasting it. It is still excellent bread, but it is difficult to metabolize for many people, especially those who are acid sensitive.

Toasting or grilling bread facilitates its digestion, because cooking cereal grains is the equivalent of predigesting them. Bread crust is more easily digested than the center portion, as the crust is more thoroughly cooked. Toasting bread slightly reduces its acidifying quality. For this same reason, crackers, which are all crust, are also less acidifying than freshly baked bread. Stale bread is less acidifying as well.

Cereal flakes that are crunchy (such as corn flakes) are less acidifying than those that are not (such as the oats used in muesli), because the former have been toasted.

The acidifying quality of pastas is typically made worse by the customary tomato sauce, tomatoes being the most acidifying vegetable. Pasta—preferably made from whole-grain flour—served plain, or with a white sauce or a little grated cheese, is a healthy alternative to pasta with tomato sauce.

Fruit pies and tarts combine several acidifying ingredients: flour, sugar, and fruit. The fruit used is often not ripe. It is better to eat such pastries only on occasion, and only when they have been made with ripe fruit. It is also a good idea to include grated or shredded almonds or cream to compensate for the acidity.

DAIRY PRODUCTS

Whole milk, whether raw or pasteurized, is alkalizing, but it becomes acidifying when it is sterilized, ultrapasteurized, homogenized, and otherwise processed, because it then becomes increasingly difficult to metabolize. Although milk is naturally alkalizing, most adults have lost the digestive capacity they had as children to make milk curdle. Milk may be safely drunk in the form of a fruit-based milkshake or smoothie, because the acidity of the fruits causes the milk to curdle in the stomach. When chocolate or sugar or both are added, milk becomes an acidifying beverage.

Cheeses with either a hard or soft crust are acidifying. Their acidity increases in proportion to their fat content, their age, and how strong they are.

Well-drained and eaten in moderation, cottage cheese and other soft unripe cheeses are slightly alkalizing. On the other hand, the more whey they contain, and the older they are, the more acid they become. (Large-curd cottage cheese tends to be better drained and thus more alkalizing than small-curd cottage cheese.) Furthermore, not only will their acidity increase, but their originally lactic levogyre L+ acids will be transformed into lactic dextrogyres D–acids. These acids are much harder to metabolize by the body, which cannot oxidize them properly because it lacks the specific enzyme necessary to transform them. The greatest part of these acids is neither assimilated nor utilized by the body but is directly eliminated in the urine in the hours immediately following their consumption. This elimination does not come without cost, however, since in order to neutralize the acidity, alkaline elements must be expended. Foods containing these kinds of lactic acids thus have a tendency to deplete the body's mineral content.

L+ lactic acid, in contrast, is very much in harmony with the body's physiology. The body transforms lactose to this form of lactic acid, and it is also what the muscles produce when burning sugar. When present in excess, L+ lactic acid causes aches and pains. The body does possess the necessary enzymes to transform L+ acid, so this substance does not have an acidifying effect.

In making yogurt, the proportion of L+ lactic acids can change completely depending on the method of fermentation used. Elevated levels of L+ lactic acid are found in the new varieties of yogurt that contain live cultures. Of course, the substantial amounts of sugar added to flavored yogurts make them acid.

Fresh butter, eaten raw and in moderation, is alkalizing, but it loses this advantage when eaten in large quantities or after being subjected to heat in cooking.

Eggs are slightly acidifying. Eaten alone, the yolk is alkalizing, however.

DAIRY PRODUCTS

Alkalizing	Slightly acidifying	Very acidifying
MILK PRODUCTS		
raw whole milk	pasteurized milk	ultrapasteurized milk
banana smoothie	fruit smoothie	chocolate milk
	crème fraîche	
BUTTER		
fresh butter		butter used in cooking (heated)
SOFT UNRIPENED CHEESES		
fresh, well drained	slightly drained	

Alkalizing	Slightly acidifying	Very acidifying
CULTURED MILK PRODUCTS		
acidophilus milk	fresh yogurt	aged yogurt
	levrogyres yogurt	dextrogyre yogurt
	(*bifidus* live culture)	sweetened yogurt with
	yogurt drinks	fruit
	without sugar	kefir
fresh whey	slightly aged whey	aged whey
fresh buttermilk		aged buttermilk
SOFT CHEESE		
	Camembert, Brie;	Same cheeses
	fresh young cheeses	but very ripe, old, with
	with little fat content	higher fat content
HARD CHEESE		
	Swiss, provolone	stronger flavored; Parmesan
EGGS		
egg yolk	whole eggs	

MEAT AND FISH

Meats can be divided into two basic groups: white and red. The latter contain a higher quantity of toxins, blood, and fat, from which their deeper color is derived. But they also have a much higher acidifying effect on the body, the worst culprit being delicatessen meats and cold cuts. Fish is not much less acidifying than meat. Crustaceans (shrimp, crayfish), however, are even more acidifying, as are the majority of shellfish. Oysters are the one exception. Their high mineral content—minerals of all sorts, not simply alkaline—makes them an excellent source of minerals for building up the body's stores.

MEAT AND FISH

Alkalizing	Slightly acidifying	Very acidifying
	MEAT	
	"white" meat: poultry, rabbit, veal, young lamb	"red" meat: beef, mutton, pork, cold cuts
	FISH	
	lean fish: whiting, sole, flounder, trout, perch	fatty fish: salmon, carp, herring, mackerel
	SEAFOOD	
oysters		crustaceans: lobster, shrimp, crayfish; mussels

LEGUMINOUS PLANTS (BEANS)

Leguminous plants are highly concentrated foods. They contain little water and consist almost entirely of proteins, lipids (fats), and glucides (carbohydrates). Peanuts, for example, contain 25 percent protein, 48 percent fat, and 25 percent glucides, leaving a mere 2 percent for water and mineral salts.

Leguminous plants are extremely potent acidifiers because of their high concentration of acidifying nutrients, and because they are rich in purines. For the body to eliminate this toxin it has to transform it into uric acid. One ounce of soybeans contains as many purines as two ounces of pork. Tofu and soy milk are much less acidifying because the process used to manufacture them makes them easier to metabolize.

LEGUMINOUS PLANTS (BEANS)

Alkalizing	Slightly acidifying	Very acidifying
SOYBEANS		
soy milk soy milk yogurt soybean sprouts	tofu	soybeans
OTHER BEANS		
	dried peas lentils kidney beans white beans navy beans	chickpeas (garbanzo beans) red beans peanuts

MISCELLANEOUS FOODS

Alkalizing	Slightly acidifying	Very acidifying
SUGAR		

raw cane sugar
  (Succanat)
pear concentrate
	maple syrup
	honey
		white and brown
		  sugar

SALT		
sea salt table salt		
SPICES AND CONDIMENTS		

green herbs:
  parsley, basil,
  etc.
		capers
		pickles
		pimentos
		mustard
		mayonnaise
		ketchup

	apple cider
	  vinegar
		other kinds of
		  vinegar

Alkalizing	Slightly acidifying	Very acidifying
	OILS	
virgin cold pressed: sunflower, olive, safflower, etc.	same oils but heat pressed	peanut, walnut, hazelnut oils used in cooking (heated)
	FATS	
nonhydrogenated vegetable margarine		hydrogenated margarine (palm or coconut oil) lard
	MUSHROOMS	
	button mushrooms	other mushrooms: truffles, morels, etc.

BEVERAGES

Water—which should be the basic drink of every human being—generally has a pH of 7, but this can vary quite a bit depending on its origins. Tap water usually has a pH of around 7. Bottled mineral waters typically have a pH of 7, but if carbonated gas is added, as is the case with many popular brands, they become acidic. Slight carbonation decreases water's normal pH of 7 to 6 or 5.5, and high carbonation decreases it even further, to 5.

The most alkaline mineral waters I have found (this is by no means an exhaustive list) are Contrexéville (France), with a pH of 7.1; Évian (France), with a pH of 7.2; Henniez bleue (Switzerland), with a pH of 7.5; and Limpia (Italy), with a pH of 7.5 (although it is officially 7.99 right at the springs). The label on the mineral water bottle will indicate the water's pH. For more information on the mineral content of waters, you can consult the Web site www.mineralwaters.org.

The water filters sold commercially to purify tap water filter out the calcium and consequently acidify the water. Nevertheless, acidification of the body's internal environment is much less dependent on consumption of water—even of slightly acid water—than it is on other factors.

Coffee, tea, and chocolate drinks are acidifying because of their purine content. Herb teas and plant-based infusions such as mint, verbena, or linden blossom are alkalizing, except for those containing rose hips, fruit peels, and birch leaves. Horsetail, like millet, is rich in silicic acid and has an acidifying effect on people whose metabolisms cannot cope with acids.

Juice made from ripe sweet fruits like mangos or peaches is alkalizing if drunk in small quantities (one small glass a day). Other juices—mainly grapefruit and orange—have an acidifying effect on individuals whose metabolisms are deficient in dealing with acids.

Vegetable juices are alkalizing as a rule, unless they are preserved by lactofermentation. Tomato juice is always acidifying, however.

As noted earlier, whey may be alkalizing or not, depending on its age.

Commercial sodas, commercial brands of lemonade, and similar beverages are very acidifying because of their high sugar content.

BEVERAGES

Alkalizing	Slightly acidifying	Very acidifying
pure water		
MINERAL WATERS		
flat with a pH of 7: Contrexéville, Évian, Henniez bleue, Limpia	slightly carbonated	heavily carbonated
TAP WATER		
depending on source and how treated	depending on source and how treated	depending on source and how treated
FILTERED WATER (CHARCOAL FILTER)		
old filter, 6.5 pH new filter, 6 pH		

COFFEE, TEA, HERB TEA

coffee substitute	green tea	coffee
mint tea, verbena,	birchbark, rose	black tea
linden, etc.	hips, fruit peels	hot chocolate
		cocoa
		horsetail

JUICE

fresh vegetables	lactofermented	tomato
fresh whey	vegetables	aged whey
almond milk	slightly aged whey	commercial lemonade,
soy milk		sodas

ALCOHOL

	beer	wine
		liqueurs, cordials
		strong spirits

Acidifying Meals and Alkalizing Alternatives

Most people choose their foods out of habit. You probably have no idea why you eat one way in preference to any other. If your eating habits are healthy, this should cause no problem. As soon as health problems appear, however, analyzing the way you eat will enable you to adjust your diet to be more balanced.

Countless people who suffer from acidification and the disorders it causes are eating highly acidifying meals without even being aware of it. The objective of this chapter is therefore to analyze the most common menus for the various meals and snack times of the day—breakfast, lunch, dinner, the ten o'clock coffee break, and the afternoon tea or snack break—to show their acidifying properties, and then to suggest some alkalizing alternatives.

The foods that make up the various menus and their suggested replacements are presented in three-column charts like those we used in the previous chapter. The columns make the same distinctions between alkalizing, slightly acidifying, and highly acidifying. It requires only a glance to determine the more or less acidifying or alkalizing nature of a meal, and of the meals suggested as healthy substitutes.

Keep in mind that the body needs foods that are naturally acidifying, such as proteins (dairy products, eggs, and so forth) and cereal grains, and that it is perfectly capable of neutralizing and eliminating their acids up to a certain point. A diet composed solely of alkaline foods is justified only if you are suffering from serious health problems brought on by acidification, and then only for a limited period. Otherwise, the diet can be gradually expanded to include more acidifying foods according to your physical ability to maintain a good acid–alkaline balance.

BREAKFAST

The three different breakfast menus provided here are among the most standard fare in contemporary culture. The replacement menus offered later in the chapter are merely suggestions or examples that can serve as guidelines. They can easily be changed and adapted according to individual need.

The conventional breakfast consists almost entirely of acidifying foods, except for butter, which is eaten in small quantity. What steps can be taken to make this meal more alkaline?

Replacing white bread with dark or whole-grain bread without yeast lowers the acidity level. The acid intake will be even less if the bread is replaced entirely by crackers or tortillas or chapatis prepared from whole-grain flour.

BREAKFAST: BREAD AND JAM

Alkalizing	Slightly acidifying	Very acidifying
	EXAMPLE	
butter		white bread
		jam or jelly
		coffee or tea with milk
		and sugar
	VARIATION 1	
butter	dark or whole-grain	
pear concentrate	bread	
coffee substitute,		
unsweetened or		
sweetened with		
natural sugar, or		
herb tea		
	VARIATION 2	
butter	dark or whole-grain	
unsweetened coffee	bread	
substitute or herb	fromage blanc, cream	
tea, or fresh	cheese	
acidophilus milk		

Jams and jellies are extremely acidifying for two reasons. First, the fruits used to make them are naturally acidic to varying degrees; and second, they typically have a very high sugar content (often as much as 50 percent).

Jelly and jam can be advantageously replaced by the pear or apple concentrates sold in health food stores. These are prepared from fruit juices that are filtered and reduced to solid form by water evaporation. They have the appearance and consistency of thin honey. These concentrates consist essentially of fructose. They have a very pleasant taste and retain a slight flavor of the fruit from which they were prepared. As they are intentionally made less acidic during the course of their preparation, they are truly alkalizing foods. Among similar products are spreads made from pears, apples, or other fruits. These are thicker and have not

71

been deacidified, so they are less alkalizing than the concentrates, but they are much more alkaline than regular jams and jellies and therefore highly preferable.

Date concentrate is another similar alkaline product.

The conventional breakfast typically includes coffee, which is extremely acidifying because of its purine content (the same is true of black tea). As decaffeinated coffee is hardly any less acidifying, you should replace it entirely with one of the numerous substitute beverages made from chicory or roasted grains. As each of these has its own unique flavor, the best solution is to try them all until you find the one that tastes best to you. The aroma and flavor of these drinks aren't exactly like coffee, but because their color, consistency, and the way they are prepared and consumed are so similar to coffee, they make great substitutes that many inveterate coffee drinkers have turned to successfully.

Tea without theine is no more a solution than decaffeinated coffee. Green tea is less acidifying than black tea, but an even better option is herb teas. Mint and verbena are well known and very popular. Rosemary, sage, and thyme have stimulant properties that can partially replace those found in coffee and tea.

To sweeten herb teas or healthy coffee substitutes, it is better to use natural sugar obtained from the whole juice of the sugar cane or a sugar that is as unrefined as possible. Because it has not been refined, it still contains all the constituent elements of the juice (vitamins, enzymes, trace elements) and consequently can be metabolized easily by the body without producing acid waste products. White sugar, as well as "brown" sugar (which is simply white sugar that has had some of the molasses that was removed during the refining process added back in), should be strictly avoided.

Best of all would be not to use sugar of any kind. It is merely a matter of breaking the habit of sweetening your beverages, because these healthy substitutes taste delicious just as they are.

Alkalizing	Slightly acidifying	Highly acidifying
	EXAMPLE	
		coffee
		croissant, muffin,
		sweet roll
	VARIATION 1	
herb tea or coffee substitute	whole-grain rusk bread (such as Melba toast) or other bread product	
	VARIATION 2	
herb tea or coffee substitute dried fruits almonds		

Coffee and a Danish, croissant, or doughnut may be all you eat for breakfast if you are in a hurry or are not hungry in the morning. Such a meal may make you feel instantly energized, but the rush of energy has not been contributed by what you've just eaten. Rather, it has been borrowed from the body's own organic reserves by the alkaloids in the coffee. Foods that can truly provide energy are rich in glucides—fresh and dried fruits, cereal grains, and potatoes. Coffee contains no glucides, unless white sugar has been added. Pastry contributes some, but they are little in quantity and poor in quality.

Coffee's lack of contribution to physical vigor is not only due to the fact that it forces the body to convert the glucides and lipids stored in the tissues into glucose. This process, which is repeated with each cup of coffee or other stimulant, overtaxes the body and leads to the production of numerous acids. These acids then combine with those brought directly into the body by the coffee itself, and sometimes with those of the orange juice that has been taken for the benefit of its vitamin C content.

This double source of acidification engenders a state of chronic fatigue. Someone who regularly uses a stimulant like coffee quickly finds himself or herself in a vicious circle. To overcome fatigue, he or she takes more of the stimulant, which only maintains the state of debilitation.

A radical change is necessary to break this vicious circle. The solution involves giving the body genuine energetic assistance with a breakfast consisting of dark bread, butter, and pear concentrate, so that it can make the transition away from the artificial stimulation provided by coffee. The coffee is gradually—but in a short period of time—eliminated from the diet and replaced by naturally stimulating beverages such as herb teas with thyme, rosemary, or sage. Grain-based or chicory beverages can substitute for the taste and appearance of coffee without replicating its stimulant qualities.

The body obviously requires some time to get used to this new menu plan, but the rewards will greatly repay all the effort necessary to stick to it.

BREAKFAST: BIRCHER MUESLI

Alkalizing	Slightly acidifying	Very acidifying
	EXAMPLE	
milk	breakfast cereal fresh fruit yogurt	
	VARIATION 1	
milk (cow or soy)	crunchy flakes	
	VARIATION 2	
cream cheese, fromage blanc dry fruit almonds	sweet, ripe fruit	

Cereal flakes are acidifying but need not be systematically eliminated from the diet, as they provide a good intake of energy for the body. Cereals are generally difficult to digest, and the poorer the digestion, the greater the problem of acidity. Untoasted or partially toasted flakes, such as are found in muesli or granola, are much harder to digest than those that have been baked or toasted to make them crunchy. In fact, the carbohydrates of cereal flakes are transformed into simpler substances by cooking. This acts as a kind of predigestion that makes digestion in the body easier. Crunchy and puffed cereals are therefore less acidifying.

There is one additional problem with cereals, and that is sugar. The sugar that is added to give a better flavor to the flakes is sometimes present in large quantity, which makes up for any reduction of the acidifying aspects by cooking. There are plenty of crunchy cereal blends, however, that have little or no sugar, or are sweetened with natural sugar or fruit juice rather than with refined white sugar.

To be digested properly, cereals need an alkaline digestive environment. Adding naturally acidic fresh fruits or yogurt to cereal upsets the digestion of the cereal and causes it to ferment, which engenders a number of acids and toxins. You can either eat cereals with milk, or eat fresh fruits with soft, unripened cheeses, such as cream cheese and fromage blanc, dried fruits, and almonds, all three of which are alkalizing.

Contrary to general belief, a blend of cereal flakes, fruits, and yogurt (or milk) does not conform to the famous muesli recipe created by Dr. Bircher.[1] His recipe used a single grain—rolled oats—in very modest helpings (one tablespoon per person), and he prescribed that the oats should be soaked overnight in water to predigest them. Although Dr. Bircher then added fresh fruits, this blend was much more digestible than the mixture known as muesli today.

Other Alkaline Breakfast Variations

Here are several additional suggestions for breakfast menus that, while they may seem a little out of the ordinary, can be quite helpful because of their alkaline character. Exclusively consisting of alkaline foods, these meals are particularly recommended for those who need to follow a very strict alkaline diet, but they are valuable for anyone simply as welcome variations on the daily meal.

OTHER BREAKFAST VARIATIONS

VARIATION 1	dried fruit
	almonds
	whey, buttermilk, or fresh white cheese
	herb tea or unsweetened coffee substitute
VARIATION 2	soaked dry fruits with soaking liquid
	fresh white cheese
	herb tea or unsweetened coffee substitute
VARIATION 3	mashed banana
	almonds or almond paste
	herb tea or unsweetened coffee substitute
VARIATION 4	chestnuts
	fresh white cheese
	herb tea or unsweetened coffee substitute

VARIATION 5	banana (or other sweet ripe fruit) smoothie made with cow's or soy or almond milk
VARIATION 6	raw carrots, raw fennel, etc.
	fresh white cheese
	unsweetened herb tea

MIDMORNING SNACK BREAK

Several hours—four to six, normally—can elapse between breakfast and lunch. To last through an entire morning with the energy necessary to get work done or complete other activities, many people absolutely require the light boost that comes from a drink and perhaps a snack.

The most common refreshments today do fulfill this goal because they are rich in glucides, the preeminent energetic source. In most cases they are also acidifying, and therefore these snacks are not recommended if you are suffering from acid–alkaline imbalance. Below are some alternate suggestions.

Alkalizing	Slightly acidifying	Very acidifying
	EXAMPLE	
sugar		coffee with sugar cookies made with white flour and sometimes with chocolate
	VARIATION 1	
coffee substitute sweetened with natural sugar	whole-grain cookies with little sugar	
	VARIATION 2	
dried fruits almonds unsweetened herb tea		
	VARIATION 3	
carrot juice		

Simply replacing pastry products or cookies made from white flour with those made from whole-grain flour, only slightly sweetened (ideally by raw cane sugar), reduces the acidifying effect of this kind of snack.

An alkaline beverage such as an herb tea or a healthy coffee substitute, which can be drunk either unsweetened or sweetened with natural sugar, should of course replace coffee (or black tea). You can also substitute crackers or cookies with dried fruits or almonds for the traditional pastry, and have an alkaline vegetable juice, such as carrot juice, for your beverage. A sensible choice of substitutes allows you to eat the kind of snack to which you are accustomed, but one with an entirely different effect on the body's acid–alkaline balance.

FRESH FRUIT SNACK

Alkalizing	Slightly acidifying	Very acidifying
EXAMPLE		
		tart apple or other tart fruit
VARIATION 1		
	sweet apple or other sweet, ripe fruit	
VARIATION 2		
dried fruits unsweetened herb tea		
VARIATION 3		
banana almonds		

Apples or other fruits are acidifying only if you have a deficiency in metabolizing acids. One option is to choose a sweet, ripe piece of fruit, which is less acidifying than less ripe, more tart fruit. There are two other options as well. The first is dried fruits—raisins, dates, bananas, and so forth—plus some almonds. The second is the only fruit that is absolutely alkaline: the banana. To be at its peak of flavor it must be completely ripe. A banana with some almonds is a delicious snack and a great alternative to the standard break-time fare.

Alkalizing	Slightly acidifying	Very acidifying
	EXAMPLE	
		ham sandwich on white bread commercial soda or lemonade
	VARIATION	
salad greens water	whole-grain bread cheese	

Commercial sodas and lemonades are very acidifying because of their high sugar content. From the dietary perspective these contain *bad sugar*; being highly refined, it enters the bloodstream rapidly and forces the pancreas to release insulin immediately to keep the blood sugar from rising too high (hyperglycemia). While this release may address the immediate crisis, the sudden and significant discharge of insulin generally causes the normal blood sugar level to drop too low, resulting in *hypo*glycemia and its consequent loss of energy. To restore the proper energy balance, the body experiences a craving for sugar. If this need is satisfied again with a bad sugar, the resulting release of more insulin eventually exhausts the pancreas, and the body's internal environment becomes acidified from the repeated intake of sugar. This in turn increases the body's demand for sugar, since the main symptom of acidification is fatigue. A vicious circle is created, similar to the one we examined with coffee. To get off this merry-go-round it is absolutely necessary to replace bad sugars (primarily white sugar and all the foods that contain it, such as soda, candy, pastry, etc.) with natural sugars: dried fruits, pear concentrate, granola bars.

Diet sodas with artificial sweeteners offer no alternative solution. Although they do not contain sugar, the ingredients normally used to replace sugar are by and large equally harmful.

Here are some more variations on the midmorning snack. The afternoon snacks outlined later in this chapter are also totally appropriate.

OTHER SNACK VARIATIONS

Alkalizing	Slightly acidifying

VARIATION 1	cream cheese, large-curd cottage cheese, or other soft white cheese sweetened with pear concentrate or natural sugar	any sweet, fully ripe fruit
VARIATION 2	Granola bars not high in sugar, no chocolate	
VARIATION 3	milk	crunchy cereal flakes
VARIATION 4	mashed banana almond paste	
VARIATION 5	almond milk	
VARIATION 6	vegetable juice	whole-grain cookies or crackers

Almond milk can be purchased in many health food stores; it can also be made by blending almond paste (available in health food stores) with a little water. This is a very flavorful, nutritious, and alkalizing beverage.

Vegetable juices (carrots, red beet, or vegetable juice cocktail) are a great source of energy because of the natural sugars they contain. Make sure the blends do not contain tomato, and that the method used to preserve them has not made them more acid (for example, lactofermentation). Keep this in mind especially if you are sensitive to acid.

LUNCH

The main meal of the day[*2] most commonly consists of a protein (in the form of meat or fish), a starch (rice, pasta, or potatoes), and vegetables (green salad or a cooked side dish). This is normally followed by coffee and dessert, or, in some cases, cheese. How does such a meal rate on the scale of acid–alkaline balance?

CLASSIC LUNCH MENU

Alkalizing	Slightly acidifying	Very acidifying
	EXAMPLE	
cooked vegetables:		red meat
carrots		sauce or gravy
green salad		white rice
		strong cheese
		white bread
		wine or soda
		sweet dessert: custard,
	pudding, cake,	
	cookies, ice cream	
		coffee with sugar
	VARIATION	
cooked vegetables:	white meat	
carrots	whole-grain cookie	
potatoes	or cake sweetened	
green salad	with natural sugar	
unsweetened herb		
tea or water		

Meat and fish are acidifying foods. It is possible to reduce their acidifying effect by choosing white meats over red and lean fish over fish with high fat content. It would be sensible to replace the meat portion of the meal every other day with eggs or cheese, as these satisfy the need for protein but in a less acidifying form. Note that the suggestion is to replace, not combine. Combining different proteins at one meal only complicates digestion and increases the acidification effect.

The fatty and flour-thickened sauces that often accompany meats have an acidifying effect; avoid them and choose grilled meat or fish instead.

Starchy foods made from grain (rice, pasta) are acidifying by nature, and even more so when refined, such as white rice or pasta made from white flour. Be careful not to overlook bread when you are analyzing this meal. Bread is acidifying, and people frequently eat quite a bit of it at lunch. Replacing bread with whole grains, such as brown rice or pasta made from whole wheat or other flours, can have a very salutary influence on the acid–alkaline balance. If this substitution does not have the desired results—as may be the case if you have a serious acidification problem—try replacing the grain-based foods with potatoes. When you are beginning a deacidification treatment, it is not really a hardship to eat potatoes on a daily basis if grain-based foods are too acidifying for your body. However, potatoes lose their alkalizing virtues if they are eaten as french fries, because the high fat content transforms them into acidifying foods.

In the lunch menus we have examined, the only truly alkalizing foods that can provide a counterbalance to the presence of acid foods are vegetables, raw or cooked. It is therefore very important to ensure that they represent a significant portion of the meal. When a piece of meat and the starch take up almost the entire surface of the plate, leaving room for only one or two spoonfuls of cooked vegetables, the role of the vegetables is no longer nutritious but merely decorative.

Sugary desserts have a double disadvantage: the additional acid intake provided directly by the sugar—most often white sugar—and the acids produced by the fermentation caused by the indigestible mixture of sugar and proteins. Cakes, pastries, custards, ice cream, and so forth are not recommended for this reason, and neither are natural fruits or fruit compotes. The ideal solution is to dispense with dessert altogether. If the urge for dessert is too strong to ignore, the best option is to limit it to simple foods: unflavored soft white cheese (cream cheese, fromage blanc), dry cookies with very little sugar, and so on.

The coffee that customarily brings the meal to a close stimulates the digestion to a slight degree, but because coffee is acidifying it is preferable to find a substitute, such as an herb tea made from nonacidifying and easily digested herbs: mint, verbena, balm, basil, rosemary, and so on.

PASTA MEALS

Alkalizing	Slightly acidifying	Very acidifying
EXAMPLE		
mixed tossed salad herbs	hot-pressed oil vinegar	spaghetti made from white flour tomato sauce Parmesan cheese
VARIATION		
mixed tossed salad virgin cold-pressed oil herbs	whole-grain pasta grated cheese, dash of vinegar or lemon juice, or yogurt	

Because of the numerous alkaline elements it contains, a generous helping of mixed salad (without tomatoes) can partially compensate for the acidifying nature of white pasta and tomato sauce. Tomatoes are well known as acidifying agents. When they are made into a sauce, their acidity increases because cooking both destroys their vitamin and mineral content and concentrates their acidic elements. When Parmesan cheese is added, the acidifying effect becomes even more intense; Parmesan is more acidic than many other cheeses, as you can tell by its taste.

Pasta-based meals can be alkalinized by using pasta made from whole-grain flour instead of refined white flour, and by eliminating the tomato sauce. Instead, eat pasta either with a little oil (virgin cold-pressed), or with some shredded cheese of a variety less acidic than Parmesan. If the idea of pasta without sauce is unthinkable, use a light white sauce or a pesto-type sauce.

It is important to keep the amount of vinegar (or lemon juice) in salad dressings small in proportion to the oil. Vinegar is highly acidic. Some people use more vinegar than oil in dressings, but many recipes call for a ratio of three parts oil to one part vinegar. The use of vinegar is so ingrained that many people find it hard to imagine a salad dressing without it. But you can create delicious salad dressings just with oil and herbs. Depending on your personal taste, soft white cheese, brewer's yeast, soy milk, vegetable juice, and so forth can also be used. The variations are endless.

If you still want a dressing that is slightly acidic, use vinegar or lemon juice, but in small doses.

The choice of oil is also important to minimize the acidifying effect of salad dressing. Choose high-quality virgin cold-pressed oil.

BEAN-BASED MEAL

Alkalizing	Slightly acidifying	Very acidifying
	EXAMPLE	
cooked vegetables	tofu	lentils, soybeans, etc.
	VARIATION 1	
cooked vegetables	whole-grain cereal tofu	
	VARIATION 2	
cooked vegetables potatoes	tofu	

A bean-based dish using lentils, soybeans, or white beans, among many others, is common in vegetarian cooking. The bean dish is usually accompanied by a vegetable (and possibly a salad), but often it contains tofu (made from soybeans) or a grain as well (rice, couscous, corn, and so on). The purpose of these combinations is not simply gastronomic but nutritional. By themselves, neither grains nor beans contain all the essential amino acids the human body needs, but combined in the right proportions, grains and beans together form a complete protein.

Leguminous plants are extremely nutritious foods, but they are also very acidifying. They are hard to digest, especially when combined with cereal grains. Poor digestion creates more acids. Unfortunately, individuals who are unable to metabolize acids properly usually also have problems with their digestive systems in general. For them, the consumption of beans and other leguminous plant foods is double jeopardy. It would be far preferable for these individuals to eat beans only on an occasional basis (for example, well-cooked lentils), and to replace beans in their diet with cereals, which are just as nutritious but much, much easier to digest. People who are sensitive to acids should eat potatoes more often than grain-based dishes, because potatoes are easy to digest and always alkaline.

The menus above offer two more alkaline variations, one with the less acidifying cereals (corn, brown rice, spelt), and the other with potatoes. Vegetarians can obtain sufficient complete protein intake by supplementing these menus with tofu.

MEALS WITH WINE

Alkalizing	Slightly acidifying	Very acidifying
EXAMPLE		
cooked vegetables potatoes	lean fish	wine
VARIATION		
cooked vegetables potatoes water	lean fish	

Composed of equal amounts of alkalizing and acidifying foods, this meal seems relatively balanced. Nonetheless, it is not advised for people suffering from acidification or for those who have trouble metabolizing acids, because of the wine. Drunk as a regular accompaniment to meals, wine generally reduces digestive capability and represents a considerable intake of acids. The alcohol it contains is neutralized by the liver, but over a long period this work exhausts the organ. Furthermore, the tannins in wine lock up the mucous membranes of the digestive tract and reduce its ability to function properly. The weaknesses this causes have an effect on the body's ability to reduce the production of acids during the digestive process. As wine is acidifying by nature, it is better to drink it only on occasion, after your acid–alkaline balance has been restored, and never when you are experiencing any sort of health problem related to acids.

The meals listed below are basic meal templates. They can be infinitely varied by changing the raw and cooked vegetable, the cheese, and so on.

OTHER MEAL VARIATIONS

VARIATION 1	Raw vegetables with sprouts
	baked potatoes
	soft white cheese
VARIATION 2	cooked vegetables
	roasted potatoes
	soft white cheese
VARIATION 3	raw vegetables with almonds
	corn polenta
	soft white cheese
VARIATION 4	corn on the cob
	soft white cheese
	cooked vegetables
VARIATION 5	green salad
	cabbage
	chestnuts
	fresh acidulated milk
VARIATION 6	green salad/raw vegetables
	potatoes
	egg yolk (hard- or soft-boiled)

The following variations are not as alkalizing as the six just presented because they all contain one acidifying food. But this food item is only slightly acidifying and represents only a small portion of the total meal, so these variations can be considered as alkaline for all practical purposes.

LESS ALKALIZING MEAL VARIATIONS

Alkalizing	Slightly acidifying

VARIATION 1	raw vegetables potatoes	Swiss-type cheese
VARIATION 2	green salad corn polenta	cheese or eggs
VARIATION 3	raw vegetables cooked vegetables chestnuts green salad butter black olives soft white cheese	cheese whole-grain crackers or dark bread
VARIATION 5	raw vegetables cooked vegetables soy sauce	fried brown rice (oriental style)
VARIATION 6	green salad cooked vegetables	grain dish (spelt, etc.) or crepes or pasta
VARIATION 7	green salad potatoes	cheese or mushroom omelet
VARIATION 8	green salad tortilla with potatoes	eggs
VARIATION 9	mixed salad cooked vegetables	tofu
VARIATION 10	green salad vegetables au gratin (with cream or milk) potatoes	cheese

MIDAFTERNOON SNACK OR TEA

Like the midmorning snack, the one in the afternoon supplies energy that bridges the gap between the previous meal and dinner. As the greatest part of the day is now past, especially that part of the day that makes up most professional activities, a natural sense of fatigue begins to make its presence felt. The reason for this is that the energy supplied by the foods eaten at lunch has been significantly depleted. Blood sugar levels are therefore low, and the need for glucides is making itself felt, often powerfully, which can drive a person to consume foods that are unhealthy and acidifying.

Sweets such as candy bars or pastries are characterized by their high refined-sugar content and usually by high levels of unhealthy fats. These products cause blood sugar levels to rise rapidly and give the body a boost with a quick supply of energy. But as we have already explained, refined sugar is one of the biggest culprits in acidification of the body.

86

SWEET SNACK

Alkalinizing	Slightly acidifying	Very acidifying
	EXAMPLE	
		chocolate candy
	VARIATION	
dried fruit: dates, figs		

A good replacement for a candy bar or pastry is dried fruit. The high natural sugar content and strong flavor make dried fruits feel filling, and the natural sugars do not trigger a hypoglycemic episode. There is a wide variety of dried fruits to choose from with many different flavors and textures, so everyone should be able to find something to his or her taste.

The chart below examines pastries, which are composed of white flour, saturated fats, and refined sugars, three ingredients that are highly acidifying. When this snack is washed down with coffee, black tea, or soda, the acidifying effects are increased.

By replacing a pastry with a whole-grain muffin sweetened with natural sugar, dried fruits, or pear concentrate, and replacing soda, coffee, or black tea with herb tea, you can lessen the acidifying effect considerably.

Pastries can also be replaced by any of a number of commercially manufactured whole-grain cookies available in the supermarket, or any other of the alkaline variations suggested in the chart. Sodas or caffeinated beverages can easily be eliminated in favor of smoothies or fruit smoothies.

PASTRY SNACK

Alkalizing	Slightly acidifying	Very acidifying
	EXAMPLE	
		pastry, black tea or soda
	VARIATION 1	
herb tea	whole-grain cake or cookies with natural sugar	
	VARIATION 2	
banana smoothie	smoothie with sweet, ripe fruit	

Fruit smoothies are not only extremely energizing thanks to their constituent fruits, but they also provide energy over a long period. The glucide (fruit)–protein (milk) blend stabilizes blood sugar levels because the proteins diminish the speed with which the body burns off the glucides and thus also acts as a brake against hypoglycemia. Smoothies can be made from regular milk or from cream cheese thinned with a little water. Soy milk can also be used. To make a smoothie, simply put the fruits and liquid in a blender and blend until smooth. If necessary, you can add a natural sweetener to taste.

The classic snack of bread with butter and/or jelly with cocoa or chocolate milk can be transformed from an acidifying meal into a more alkalizing one simply by a more judicious selection of its components. By choosing dark or whole-grain bread over white, substituting a natural sweetener like pear concentrate for jelly, and replacing the cocoa or chocolate milk with herb tea or plain milk, you have changed this snack into a completely alkalizing meal.

BREAD AND JAM SNACK

Alkalizing	Slightly acidifying	Very acidifying
	EXAMPLE	
butter		white bread
		jam or jelly
		hot chocolate
		or chocolate milk
	VARIATION	
butter	dark or whole-grain	
pear concentrate	bread	
herb tea or milk		

Fruits and fruit juices do not have the same acidifying effects on everyone. They have been classified among the acidifying foods because this book is primarily directed toward people whose metabolisms are deficient in dealing with acids. For these individuals, yogurt, which is naturally acid, can be replaced by soft white cheese or fresh acidophilus milk, and fresh fruits by dried fruits such as bananas or raisins, which, if they have been soaked beforehand, go better with the soft white cheese.

FRUIT SNACK*

Alkalizing	Slightly acidifying	Very acidifying
	EXAMPLE	
	sweet, ripe fruit	tart fruit or fruit juice
	fresh yogurt	aged yogurt
	VARIATION	
dried fruit		
soft white cheese		

*A midafternoon snack serves exactly the same purpose as a midmorning snack, so these meals are easily interchangeable. Any alkaline variation suggested for the midmorning snack would work just as well here.

Dinner for some people is the big meal of the day and uses the same types of menus as the standard lunch meals we examined earlier. For other people, dinner is a much smaller affair. Despite its straightforward appearance, it is often much more complicated and much more acidifying than you might think. This is especially true for the evening meal composed of bread with butter and jelly or cold cuts and cheese, and coffee—a repast that is common because it requires little preparation.

We now understand the acidifying nature of coffee, bread, and jelly. Cold cuts and cheese as high-protein foods are also highly acidifying, but cold cuts are much more so because of their greater concentration of saturated fats. On the digestive level, it is not so simple, and it is even more complex on the level of acid–alkaline balance. In fact, when a meal of this kind is composed totally of acidifying foods, the body is forced to neutralize the acids it ingests solely with the alkaline substances it draws from its own tissues.

To restore balance to this kind of meal, include a generous helping of green salad or raw vegetables. Rather than drink coffee, pick another beverage such as herb tea; or, best of all, vegetable soup, which is rich in alkaline substances. By replacing white bread with whole-wheat or other whole-grain bread and strong cheese with milder cheese, you can lower the acid levels of this kind of meal even further.

LIGHT SUPPER OR LUNCH

Alkalizing	Slightly acidifying	Very acidifying
	EXAMPLE	
butter	cheese	white bread
	honey	cold cuts
		strong cheese
		jam or jelly
		coffee
	VARIATION	
green vegetables	whole-grain bread	
or raw vegetables	or crackers	
or vegetable soup	cheese	
herb tea	honey	

Pies and fruit tarts are acidifying because of their combination of ingredients. The fruits used for making pies are often unripe and call for additional sugar.

Furthermore, the combination of starch (pastry crust) and a weak-acid food (fruits) upsets the digestion and allows fermentation to occur, encouraging the production of acids.

There are no good alternatives to fruit tarts or pies. If you are suffering from acidification and crave such foods, you should simply be aware of their nature and consequences and limit your intake. However, a less acidic variation can be made from unrefined flour, a natural sugar, and fully ripened fruits.

FRUIT PIES AND TARTS

Alkalizing	Slightly acidifying	Very acidifying
	EXAMPLE	
		pastry crust
		fruits
		white sugar
	VARIATION	
	pastry crust from unrefined flour	
	natural sugar	
	fully ripened fruits	

Pizza is an extremely acidifying food because of its principal ingredients. Two alternatives are possible, but neither includes tomatoes, which are always acidifying. The first is a vegetable pie. The acidification effects can be made less significant by the vegetables and a crust made from unrefined, whole-grain flour. The second alternative is a cheese pizza. It is not truly an alkalizing food, but its slightly acidifying nature can be diminished even further if it is accompanied by a large green salad or a generous helping of raw vegetables.

PIZZA

Alkalizing	Slightly acidifying	Very acidifying
EXAMPLE		
mozzarella cheese black olives	whole-grain pizza crust grated cheese	white flour pizza crust tomatoes or tomato sauce
VARIATION 1		
pizza with vegetable toppings	whole-grain pizza crust grated cheese	
VARIATION 2		
green salad	pizza with cheese whole-grain pizza crust grated cheese	

In addition to the other alkaline variations that were already listed as lunch suggestions, vegetable soup is another evening meal possibility.

Vegetable soup offers a countless number of possibilities for varied meals. With a simple change of ingredients you can create a limitless range of soups that look and taste entirely different from one another. Be careful, however, not to thicken soups with cereal-based starches; use potatoes instead. When accompanied by a little cheese (to provide protein) and possibly some whole-grain bread, soup is a very pleasant meal, especially during the cold months of the year.

Part Three

NEUTRALIZING AND ELIMINATING ACIDS

Drinking large amounts of water on a daily basis can be a very effective way to deacidify the body. Our bodies need a lot of water to function properly and to eliminate acids; water drunk in large quantities, if it is alkaline, can neutralize numerous acids.

WATER AND THE PRODUCTION AND ELIMINATION OF ACIDS

The body's substance is less solid than we may think. Solids represent only 30 percent of total body weight, which means our bodies are 70 percent water!

This water forms blood, lymph, extracellular fluid (the fluid that surrounds the cells), and intracellular fluid (the liquid inside the cells). Water is present in such large quantity inside the body because it constitutes the environment of the cells. Our cells live in an aquatic environment, swimming in an ocean of liquid that both surrounds and fills them with water.

The body should therefore always be well hydrated, so that the cells have enough water at their disposal to function properly. Ideal hydration permits not only the cells but also the enzymes to work in an optimum manner; in fact, it is only when the enzymes are working well that the cells can do their jobs.

Enzymes are the little "workers" responsible for a large number of biochemical transformations that are necessary to physical function. Digestion, assimilation, growth, tissue repair, elimination, energy production, and more all depend on the activity of enzymes.

As is the case for all living things, enzymes require a healthy environment to conduct their activities. They must have enough space and a sufficient quantity of water, the principal vital element of their environment, at their disposal to fulfill their mission. When the body lacks water, the enzymes cannot work as effectively.

When we do not drink enough, the body becomes dehydrated. The volume of cellular fluids shrinks, and the substances the fluids contain, as well as the enzymes, are more tightly packed together. Body fluids that are highly concentrated provide an unfavorable environment for enzymatic activity, and the quality of this environment continues to deteriorate as the dehydration worsens.

First the enzymes slow their working rhythm. Later, this rhythm becomes even slower; biochemical transformations are poorer and fewer in number. Instead of being carried through to completion, the transformations are interrupted at intermediate stages. At these intermediate stages—and this is of the utmost importance for the subject of this book—the transformed substances are most often in an acid state. Pyruvic acids, succinic acids, and others result from the poor transformation of sugars; cetonic acids, from the poor transformation of fats; and so on. When the body is dehydrated, it becomes acidified with substances it has created itself.

Most people think of dehydration as the severe, acute kind that occurs when travelers are lost in the desert without water and die in a day or two. But there is also chronic dehydration, which is not as abrupt or intense. *Chronic dehydration is very widespread at present and affects everyone who does not drink enough liquids to meet his or her body's needs.*

The troubles chronic dehydration cause are not as pronounced as those created by the acute form. The lack of fluid is not substantial enough to cause death or serious illness, but it is still enough to generate numerous functional disorders, such as acidification of the internal cellular environment, with all the health problems that can result.

Another reason why the lack of water contributes to the acidification of the body is that the constituent fluids of the body transport the wastes manufactured on the cellular level, including acid wastes, to the organs responsible for waste elimination, such as the skin and kidneys.

The intracellular fluid is the first to transport the acids. The acids are brought to the external membrane of the cell so they can cross through it into the extracellular fluid, which then relays the acids to a capillary vessel. Crossing through the vessel's thin walls, the acids are carried by the bloodstream to an excretory organ.

Chronic dehydration reduces the volume of these bodily fluids, which become thicker and less fluid; their capacity for circulating and transporting wastes diminishes. The acids stagnate in the tissues instead of being eliminated, and as they accumulate, they acidify the body.

The support media in which acids are evacuated by the excretory organs are also fluids. The kidneys and the sweat glands are the two main excretory organs used for the evacuation of acids. The urine excreted by the kidneys is 95 percent water; sweat is 99 percent water. A scarcity of water forces the body to reduce the volume of liquid—and hence of the waste acids—that it excretes as urine and sweat to avoid creating greater dehydration. But the body can reduce the amount of liquid used for elimination purposes only so far. If urine becomes too concentrated, its flow is inhibited, and the fluid becomes too harsh for the delicate mucous membranes of the urinary system.

Acids that are not being eliminated in sufficient quantity remain inside the body and contribute to its acidification.

An excretory organ that lacks enough liquid to eliminate acids is like a stream whose flow has become too slow. The sand and other debris it carries are no longer pulled along by the current but are deposited in the stream bed and on its banks. All it needs is an increased flow of water for all these deposits to be carried away.

One of the means of fighting acidification, then, is to drink large quantities of water every day. But how much water should you drink?

Every day we eliminate something on the order of 2.5 liters of water. This includes 1.5 liters of urine, 0.5 liter of sweat, 0.4 liter through the lungs, and 0.1 liter in the stools. It makes sense to think that we should put 2.5 liters of water a day back into the body to compensate for these losses and avoid establishing a deficiency. This volume should not include only liquids ingested as drinks, because food also imports water into the body. Fruits and vegetables contain around 90 percent water, meats 70 percent, cheeses 30 to 50 percent, cereal grains 11 percent, and so forth. According to the World Health Organization, drinking 2 liters of water a day should be sufficient.

This figure should really be higher, though, because of our current diet and lifestyle. Various factors can increase the body's need for water: foods that are too salty, rich, and concentrated; as well as alcohol, tobacco, and overeating in general, as it requires more water to dilute the toxins these foods bring into the body. Stress, excessively vigorous exercise, overheated buildings, and so forth also increase water needs, because in these conditions the body sweats more.

An adequate water intake to keep the body well hydrated, therefore, is 2.5 to 3 liters of water a day. The vast majority of people, however, never drink this much; typical consumption tends to fall below the World Health Organization's suggested 2 liters daily. Many people find it impossible to drink 2 to 3 liters of water a day, but it is really only a matter of making it a habit. They might also say that they are not thirsty, but lack of thirst is characteristic of chronically dehydrated people. In their case, the absence of the sensation of thirst does not mean the body has all the water it needs. Rather, because this alarm signal has been ignored, a water deficiency no longer triggers it. The signal will reappear, however, once these people start drinking more.

While the benefits conferred by simply drinking 2 to 3 liters of water a day with regard to acidification are significant in their own right, there is an even greater advantage when the water is alkaline. We now take a look at this qualitative aspect of water.

ALKALINE WATER AND DEACIDIFICATION

What are the available waters, and what is their pH?

The drinking water nature provides is primarily spring water, but there is not enough spring water to supply the needs of the ever-growing population of planet Earth, so we must turn to other sources, such as underground aquifers, rivers, and lakes. The water from these sources first needs to be cleaned and disinfected. It also needs to be treated, most often with chlorine, so that it will not be altered by a prolonged stay in the pipes that carry it to the consumer. The tap water obtained in this way doesn't have the same qualities as spring water, although an attempt is made to render it as similar as possible. This goal is partially realized from the chemical point of view, but not always. In any case, it is not often achieved from the standpoint of taste, because the chlorine gives water an unpleasant odor and flavor.

As a remedy for these annoyances, more and more people purify their drinking water with filters. The elimination of chlorine, excess mineral content (calcium), toxic metals like lead, or organic residues (nitrates) can be achieved with carafe filters or more sophisticated devices like reverse-osmosis filters. Another way to handle this is to purify water through distillation.

The pH of spring water varies from one spring to the next depending on the spring's mineral composition. This pH is indicated on the labels of the bottles in which spring waters are sold. Tap water is neutral or slightly alkaline, but this too depends on the nature of the water at its original source. Depending on the effectiveness of the filter, filtered waters have a pH that ranges from neutral to acid. This is also true for distilled water. The reason is that filters strip the water of the minerals it contains, primarily calcium, magnesium, and sodium, which are responsible for a water's alkalinity, so these waters tend to be acidic.

It is possible to deacidify the internal cellular environment with water from alkaline mineral springs. Tap water can work, but because it is hardly alkaline or neutral, its therapeutic effects are weak. Filtered water and distilled water, used as they are, do not help alkalinize the body's internal cellular environment because they are most often acidic. They can be made alkaline, however, by treating them with special commercially available preparations.

These preparations contain alkaline minerals like potassium, magnesium, or calcium in a form that is particularly easy for the body to assimilate. They are basically mineral solutions you mix into the water you intend to drink.

The concentration of these solutions is quite high; it only requires a few drops to alkalinize one liter of water to pH 9.5 or higher, making the treated water around 500 times more alkaline than water with a pH of 7. Another significant advantage of these drops is that they add practically no taste or odor to the water, so it remains quite pleasant to drink.

By drinking 2 or 3 liters of distilled water, filtered water, or tap water treated with an alkaline solution, we can bring into the body numerous alkaline substances for neutralizing the acids. Along with an alkaline diet, it is one of the best methods for restoring the acid–alkaline balance.

A water with a pH of 9.5 or higher is rarely if ever found in nature. The natural water supplied by rain or rivers has a pH that borders on 7.5. Water that has been made alkaline with these special drops is therefore not intended to be a permanent replacement for normal water. This is therapeutic water that should be used only for treatments over a limited period. Treatments can extend over a period of months, even a year or two, but once the acid–alkaline balance has been restored, you should resume drinking water that is closer to what nature has to offer.

There is no need to be concerned that the high alkalinity of these waters will neutralize the acidic gastric juices and hamper the digestive processes, or conversely, that the acidity of the gastric juices will neutralize the alkalinity of this water and make it ineffective in deacidification. Of course, ingested during the course of a meal, water this alkaline serves as a buffer to the acids of the gastric juices; this is why it is not advised to drink it while eating. But throughout the rest of the day, in between mealtimes, the stomach is not secreting acids, and the alkaline minerals provided by the water are entirely available for the body's use.

This doesn't change the fact that this water must be properly assimilated. You might think that all water is the same, and that one kind of water is just as easy to assimilate as any other. Yet this is not at all the case. Different waters have very different properties. Some are much more easily absorbed by the body; it all depends on their degree of structuring.

Water molecules do not remain side by side as isolated entities but gather in masses of varying sizes. If the molecules form large masses, it makes the water less fluid. To employ scientific terminology, we would say that the water is barely structured and has a high surface tension.

A highly structured water, on the other hand, which means water consisting of small masses of water molecules, is very fluid. It divides and disperses easily and spreads out better than water consisting of large masses. Because of their reduced size, these masses can cross through the body's cell membranes and mucous membranes (such as those of the digestive tract) easily and rapidly; this makes the water they form very assimilable and hydrating.

Easy assimilation of water is very important; it is futile to drink copious amounts of alkaline water on a daily basis if the alkaline minerals in the water cannot be easily assimilated.

What defines a water as being highly structured? Its structure is proportionate to its richness in varied trace elements, which is high in the case of the waters nature provides. It is around these trace elements that the masses of water molecules form. Water distilled or purified by reverse osmosis, in contrast, no longer contains the minerals around which the water molecules can collect in groups, so it is not highly structured. It is the latter kind of water that alkaline preparations are designed to be used with.

The commercially available preparations for structuring water contain more than seventy different trace elements and minerals in solution. Adding several drops to a quart of drinking water gives the water a solid structure. The capacity of structured water to penetrate the tissues ensures that the body is much better hydrated.

As we have seen at the beginning of this chapter, good hydration is an important factor for the reduction of acid production and facilitates the elimination of acids. There is thus a double advantage to drinking large quantities of water every day.

7

Alkaline Supplements

While the adoption of an alkaline diet can interrupt the acidification process and reduce the concentration of acids in the body, diet alone is not sufficient to completely remove excess acids from the body's internal environment. The reformed diet needs the reinforcement of alkaline supplements.

The greatest problem for people suffering from acidification is not the presence of acids circulating on the surface—in the bloodstream, for example—but the concentrated mass of acids that has accumulated in the deep inner tissues. *How did these acids get there in the first place?*

Blood does not contain great amounts of acid. Because the pH of blood must stay within a narrow range, the body seeks to remove acids from the bloodstream as rapidly as possible.

In addition to the neutralization of acids by the body's buffer system, the body has two other means for disposing of them. The first, which is also the most beneficial, is the elimination of acids through urine and sweat, which keeps the acids from dangerously altering the healthy pH level of the blood.

Unfortunately, the quantities of acids that have built up are often beyond the ability of the skin and kidneys to deal with effectively. The body is then forced to use a second option to protect the integrity of the blood pH. This consists of directing the acids not to the organs of elimination, which would discharge them, but into the tissues, which can withstand fluctuations of pH levels better than the blood. For people whose lifestyle and diet are highly acidifying, and for those who are metabolically deficient in dealing with acids, this repression process is constant. As each new ingestion of acids forces the previous acids a little deeper into the tissues, the amount of acids that builds up can be considerable.

The deacidification of the body, or the correction of an acidified internal environment, therefore requires the neutralization and elimination of a very large quantity of acids. It might seem that an intensive, sustained period of cleansing would allow all this built-up acid to be eliminated by stimulating the skin and kidneys to free the body of these toxins. Unfortunately, this is not the case.

To reach the skin and kidneys, the acids embedded in the tissues must first enter the bloodstream, which then carries them to the renal and subcutaneous filtering systems. This is where the difficulty lies, as the blood cannot take in much acid at one time without risking too great a deviation from its normal pH level, endangering the smooth operation and even the survival of the entire body.

The blood, therefore, accepts only minimal quantities of acid at a time and prevents any excess from entering, which strongly reduces the possibility of eliminating the acids through the skin and kidneys. To address this situation, the acids can be made to enter the blood in an altered form that causes them to lose their acid characteristics. This form is that of a neutral salt, which is obtained by the addition of an alkaline substance. An acid and alkaline combined form a neutral salt.

To neutralize each acid you want removed from the body you need a corresponding alkaline substance, but the elimination routes do not supply such substances. Alkalines brought in by an alkaline diet, even a strict one, are often not enough to do the job or would require far too much time (years) to perform it efficiently. The change in diet is primarily meant to deal with the body's current need for alkaline substances, not for disposing of the previous accumulation of acids. It is therefore imperative to provide alkaline substances in addition to those the body is ingesting through food. This is possible with alkaline supplements, preparations containing the principal alkaline minerals—calcium, potassium, magnesium, and so forth—in a form that is easily assimilated by the body.

Taking these alkaline supplements on a regular basis supports the body's efforts and greatly accelerates the process of deacidification. The supplements also provide quicker relief to the patient experiencing the painful symptoms or harmful disorders caused by excess acids in the body. Thanks to supplements, these disorders diminish, often in a remarkably short period.

The disappearance of symptoms and superficial disorders does not mean that the body has gotten rid of all its acids. They still remain in the deeper tissue layers, but the reduction in their concentration causes an initial disappearance of the minor problems that their presence may cause. Later, if this kind of supplemental therapy is maintained for a sufficient period, the internal environment is cleansed of all the acids that have built up and is therefore able to return to its normal functioning. The state of total health reached in this way can then be maintained without taking alkaline supplements but simply by adopting the appropriate lifestyle and following an adequate diet.

There are more than a dozen different kinds of alkaline supplements available today, whereas twenty years ago there were only three or four. This increase is due to the growing public awareness of the health problems caused by acid–alkaline imbalance.

This diversity offers a great advantage because, although the supplements are all fundamentally similar, their differences and individual features allow their use to be adapted to the widely varying needs of a greater number of individuals.

The following analysis focuses on twelve products. It is by no means exhaustive, but examines supplements with which the author has personal experience. Names of distributors of these and similar products available in the United States are provided in the Resources section. All these products are of proven effectiveness. They are listed not in order of effectiveness or preference but alphabetically. If readers know of alkaline supplements that are not mentioned here, they can easily evaluate them using the criteria outlined later in the chapter.

The twelve products are Alcabase, Alkala, Basa Vita, Basin, Equilibre-Vital, Erbasit, Flügge's Alkaline Blend, Ideal Base Plus, Megabase, pHion Blue, Probase, and Rebasit. (See summary chart; for information on where to obtain Erbasit and pHion Blue please see the Resources section at the end of this book.)

In the section that follows, we look at the composition of these alkaline supplements, how much of them to take and when (dosage), and the length of time they should be taken.

COMPOSITION OF ALKALINE SUPPLEMENTS

The majority of these preparations contain five alkaline minerals: calcium, potassium, magnesium, iron, and manganese. To make a supplement with only one of these minerals would be a mistake, because the body's needs are well defined, and too large a dose of any mineral can surpass the body's capacity to assimilate it. Furthermore, the body's buffer system makes use of all these minerals, each of which has a specific reason to be included in these combinations.

The Five Base Minerals

Calcium (Ca) is the mineral with the greatest presence in the human body. It is found mainly in the skeleton, but it is an indispensable part of many of the other tissues, primarily those that make up the nervous system. Potassium (K) plays a fundamental role in cellular exchanges. If there is a deficiency of this mineral, the body's energy production is poor, and muscle cramps occur. Magnesium (Mg) is well known for its calming effect on the nervous sytem and its stimulating effect on the immune system. Iron (Fe) is necessary to carry oxygen in the blood, which is of critical importance for people who have trouble metabolizing acids, since, among other deficiencies, they cannot oxidize volatile acids properly. Manganese (Mn) acts as a catalyst in numerous biochemical reactions.

If these minerals are to be of optimum benefit, it is very important that the proportion of each one in the combination is carefully chosen. In fact, the use of different nutrients by the body depends on the subtle balances between these minerals. For example, too high a presence of one can act like a brake on the assimilation of another, or the lack of one may prevent a second from being used, even if it is available in large quantity.

There are some slight variations in the ingredients of the different alkaline supplements described here, but all are balanced. However, some do not contain all five of the minerals listed (for example, the Alkala preparation does not contain iron, magnesium, or manganese; the Flügge base blend does not contain either potassium or iron; and the Megabase blend is missing both manganese and iron). Blends of this nature should be chosen when for one reason or another you need to restrict intake of one or more of these minerals.

Presence or Absence of Sodium (Na)

Sodium is a mineral used in great quantities by most people on a daily basis, as it is found in ordinary salt in the form of sodium chloride. The principal property of salt is the retention of water in the tissues. One gram of salt will retain 11 grams of fluid.

Consequently, excess sodium results in general or local edema (such as swollen ankles or fingers). When the tissues are swollen, blood pressure can rise dangerously high (hypertension) and put strain on the heart, causing it to tire. The kidneys may also deteriorate prematurely from overwork, because they are responsible for eliminating sodium excess.

An excess of sodium in the tissues can be corrected by either reducing the intake of salt or by increasing intake of potassium, which is the antagonist of sodium.

While excessive sodium in the body has a tendency to raise blood pressure and is generally stimulating, a sodium deficiency results in hypotension and apathy.

Among the alkaline supplements listed, two do not contain sodium: Basa Vita and pHion Blue. Although equally effective when it comes to neutralizing acids, these blends are especially recommended for individuals who want to deacidify but who also suffer from water retention, edema, or heart or kidney problems.

On the other end of the spectrum, the Rebasit preparation has a very high sodium content (74 percent), which makes it unsuitable for anyone suffering from the problems just mentioned. It is, however, recommended for people with low blood pressure or who lack vitality and muscle tonicity. All the other supplements listed contain modest quantities of sodium, which, furthermore, are always combined with its antagonist, potassium.

Silica

Silica is an acid mineral, as it appears in the form of silicic acid. Its presence in alkaline supplements is easily explained. Silica is of great help in a large number of the disorders that affect acidified people, including hair loss, fragile nails, dental cavities, skin problems, and joint pains. The soundness of the skeletal frame, teeth, nails, and hair, as well as the suppleness of the skin, depend in large part on silica.

Six of the alkaline blends listed contain this important mineral: Alkala, Basa Vita, Erbasit, Flügge, Megabase, and Rebasit. Silica does not have an acidifying effect when ingested in these preparations because it is present in very small quantities, whose acidity is neutralized by the large amounts of alkaline substances with which it is combined. Its benefits can thus be obtained without causing more acidification.

This is not the case with the silica found in horsetail and millet, which are often recommended for combatting disorders caused by mineral depletion, because their content of this mineral is much higher than that of the alkaline supplement blends.

Other Minerals

Several minerals (copper, strontium, and vanadium) are used in the preparation of the supplement Basin, but not in any other. These minerals do not play a major role in the body's buffer system, but they can contribute to restoring the acid-alkaline balance because of their specific properties. Copper, for example, is essential for forming red corpuscles, so it is important in the transport of oxygen and the acids dependent upon it. The roles played by strontium and vanadium are not clear. The product pHion Blue contains phosphorous for a better absorption of calcium

Form of the Supplements

The minerals contained in these alkaline supplements must be in a form the body can metabolize properly. In the blends listed they are most often prepared as salts, meaning combinations of an acid and a base. But the acids used for this purpose are weak and easily oxidized, so the body can get rid of them quickly, leaving the alkaline substance behind. The majority of blends consist of citrates—alkaline salts with a weak-acid component—whose acidic portion is easily oxidized and expelled from the body by the lungs. Other forms of alkaline mineral blends are carbonates, tartrates, sulfates, gluconates, and lactates.

Preparations containing weak acids can show an acid pH reading on litmus paper. This in no way means that these products have an acidifying effect, because the acid portion of the salts absorbed by the body is rapidly eliminated, even by people who have a metabolic deficiency in handling acids.

Whey

Whey is well known for its cleansing qualities. It stimulates renal elimination (diuretic effect), intestinal elimination (laxative effect), and elimination by the liver. It therefore encourages the elimination of toxins in general, including acids.

Whey is also rich in minerals, most of them alkaline, which makes it an excellent source for restoring minerals to the body—potassium in particular, as whey is exceptionally rich in this substance (2 percent).

When combined with alkaline blends, whey is therefore doubly useful, as it encourages elimination and restores mineral content to the body. One product contains whey: Basa Vita.

People who are allergic to milk sugar or who are lactose intolerant should not take products containing whey.

Medicinal Plants

Plants with medicinal properties have also been added to certain blends. Anise and wormwood, like wood charcoal, stimulate the digestive processes and fight intestinal fermentation (Megabase). Erbasit contains elder, linden, fennel, chamomile, and marigold, plants that have beneficial effects on both digestion and elimination, providing additional support to the deacidification process.

Product	Ca	K	Mg	Fe	Mn	Na	Si	Others	Whey	Medicinal plants	Taste	Powder	Tablets
Alcabase	•	•	•	•	•	•					salty or lemony	•	•
Alkala	•	•	•	•	•	•					salty	•	
Basa Vita	•	•	•	•	•	•					orange	•	
Basin	•	•	•	•	•	•		Cu, Va, St	•		salty	•	
Equilibre-Vital	•	•	•	•	•	•					broth		•
Erbasit	•	•	•	•	•	•	•			elder	orange	•	•
Flügge	•	•	•	•	•	•	•				salty	•	
Ideal Base Plus	•	•	•	•	•	•		vit. B_1, B_2, B_6, PP, Inositol, Zn			salty	•	•
Megabase	•	•	•	•	•	•	•			anise, absinthe, wood charcoal	anise	•	
pHion Blue	•	•	•	•	•			P			lemony	•	•
Probase	•	•	•	•	•	•		Zn			salty	•	•
Rebasit	•	•	•	•	•	•	•				salty	•	

Other Additives

Other natural substances in these alkaline mineral blends, such as malt or dextrin, are used simply as binding agents and have negligible effects on health. One exception is the natural brewer's yeast, an energy booster, in the combination Basinette.

Taste

The taste of alkaline supplements is important. A therapy using one of these supplements can last for months. Persevering and sticking to a regular schedule are much easier if the taste of the product is agreeable.

Some of these preparations have a neutral flavor with a more or less salty accent from the different salts used in their manufacture (Alcabase, Alkala, Basin, Flügge, Ideal Base Plus, Probase, Rebasit). Some products are flavored with fruit pulp. Alcabase and pHion Blue have a lemony taste, and Erbasit and Basa Vita are flavored with orange. The Megabase product has an anise flavor, but the most distinctive flavor is that of Equilibre-Vital, which tastes like broth.

Alkaline supplements are available in powdered form, to be blended with water, or in tablet form, to be swallowed with a glass of water.

ALKALINE SUPPLEMENT INTOLERANCE

Except for the warning given earlier about preparations containing large quantities of sodium, generally speaking alkaline supplements are very easily tolerated. They can on occasion cause intestinal gas and mild diarrhea at the beginning of a treatment. Most often this is not due to an intolerance for these substances, but is a temporary manifestation of taking too much initially before the body has had time to adjust.

The solution to this problem is to start with small doses and gradually increase the quantity being taken. If discomfort persists, it is probably because an ingredient in the blend is not suitable for the individual in question. In that case, a different blend should set everything right.

ALKALINE SUPPLEMENT DOSAGES

In contrast to most remedies, alkaline supplements have no fixed dosage instructions. The dosage always depends on the individual, so you are responsible for figuring out which dose is correct for your needs.

To determine the right dosage, it is of fundamental importance to take as much of an alkaline supplement as necessary to obtain a urinary pH reading that falls between 7 and 7.5.

Because many people are unaware of or ignore this rule of thumb, they do not gain maximum benefit from this therapy. The reason for taking alkaline supplements is to supply the body with its daily alkaline requirements so as to neutralize the acids that saturate its tissues. Of course, this quantity varies from one person to the next, just as the degree of acidification is not the same for everyone.

When the dosage is too low to meet the body's needs, neutralization of acids still occurs, but to a much smaller degree than could have been achieved, so the treatment does not live up to expectations. The treatment also takes much longer and is never complete, because the body still lacks enough alkaline substance to detoxify the deep tissues of their acids.

The purpose of alkaline supplement–based therapies is to neutralize and eliminate not only surface acids, but also those that have built up in the depths of the body's internal environment, until they have all been removed and optimum health has been restored. It is only at this point that the body is completely detoxified of acid wastes. This is a real cure, not simply superficial improvement of symptoms. In fact, the true nature of the condition is not its surface symptoms but the toxic state of the body's internal environment when saturated with acid wastes.

To determine the appropriate individual dosage levels of the alkaline supplement you have chosen, first take a series of urinary pH readings to determine the average value. For four to five days, measure urinary pH with the litmus paper and record the results on a suitable chart (see the sample and the "Urinary pH Record" chart). This should be long enough to allow a clear indication of your average pH. To see the effect of the supplement, continue taking the urinary pH as you begin the treatment.

For example, let's say you have a urinary pH that is more or less 5 throughout the day. A pH reading of 5 is acid, even highly acid, a sign of an acidified internal environment. To detoxify this acidic state, an alkaline supplement is definitely called for. To determine the ideal dosage, begin with small doses and gradually increase them until the urinary pH reaches 7 to 7.5.

Start with a level teaspoon of powder mixed with water and take it before each of the three main meals of the day. If the urinary pH rises to 6, increase the next day's dosage to a heaping rather than a level teaspoonful of powder three times a day. If this increase results in a pH of 7 to 7.5, you can maintain this dosage for the duration of the therapy. If the urinary pH remains below 7, you need to increase the dosage further—to 2 heaping teaspoonfuls before each meal, or even three.

Do not worry about taking too much. If you have to take a significant amount to bring the urinary pH to 7 to 7.5, it is because your body needs it.

Once you have determined the proper dosage for the duration of the therapy by this means, there is no longer any need to take daily readings of urinary pH.

People suffering from acidification whose urine is alkaline cannot use urinary pH readings as a basis for determining the proper dosages of alkaline supplements. They should start with an average dose and try to guide themselves according to whether their symptoms get better or worse.

As the therapy progresses, the acids that have built up in the body are neutralized and eliminated. As their concentration gradually diminishes, so too does the body's need for alkaline products to neutralize them. After a certain period the dosage that was necessary at the beginning of the therapy may be too high for the body's new requirements.

Therefore, once-a-month readings of urinary pH should be taken over a one- to two-day period. As long as the pH remains between 7 and 7.5, continue taking the supplement at its current dosage. If the reading is below 7—if it is 6.5 or lower—increase the dosage. This is rarely necessary, however. More often than not, after several weeks or months (some treatments may require a year or two) the pH climbs to 8 or higher. This means the body no longer requires as much alkaline material as before and is getting rid of the excess in the urine, which naturally becomes more alkaline. At this point you can reduce the dosage until the urinary pH again reads between 7 and 7.5. In this way the body receives exactly what it requires to correct its internal environment.

This kind of dosage readjustment should be performed on a regular basis over the course of the therapy. In this way, the quantity of the alkaline supplements in the diet will gradually diminish.

LENGTH OF TREATMENT

Alkaline supplement therapies are undertaken for as long as the body needs them to clear up the acid toxification of its internal environment. This varies from one individual to the next. It can last anywhere from six months to two years, based on the degree of acidification. This may seem like a long time, but it is quite short when you consider that the body was building up these acid waste deposits for a good number of years before any health problems appeared.

The sign that the therapy has reached its goal and can now be stopped is when you have a urinary pH of 7 to 7.5 without taking any alkaline supplements. This value appears naturally because the further the treatment progresses, the greater the reduction in the need for alkaline supplements. One day, following the monthly pH reading, the small amount of alkaline supplements you are still taking can be eliminated.

Of course, it is only the alkaline supplement–based therapy that you stop, not the alkaline diet that you have been following in parallel. You must maintain the diet to conserve all you have gained with the therapy. If you abandon the diet, acidification of the body picks up anew, and all your old health problems reappear.

The strictness of this alkaline diet depends on the physical capacities of each individual to metabolize acids properly. It remains quite strict for those who have trouble metabolizing acids, but most people have much greater leeway. In all cases the soundness of the diet can be determined through urinary pH. If it becomes acid again, the diet has become too expansive.

At the end of an alkaline supplement treatment the body is thoroughly cleansed of acid wastes. This is reflected by a long-forgotten state of vitality and well-being. Many people have said they never realized how good one could feel when one is healthy!

If your ability to metabolize acids properly is poor, the diet necessary to maintain a urinary pH of 7 to 7.5 would be so strict that not only would it be impossible to follow but it would probably create other deficiencies. In fact, the intake of proteins and grains would be so limited that the body could not obtain all the nutrients it needs.

If you have this particular metabolic deficiency, you should not attempt to follow a diet that is perfect in theory but unrealizable in practice. Instead, include a degree of variety in your diet and compensate for any excess acids by continuing to take alkaline supplements. Under certain circumstances, this is the only means of dealing with the physical deficiency while maintaining a diet and lifestyle that are physiologically and psychologically acceptable.

8

Other Important Supplements

In addition to the alkaline minerals mentioned in the previous chapter, there are other supplements that are quite useful for deacidifying the body: green food, enzyme supplements, prebiotic and probiotic complexes, and antioxidant complexes. All four reduce the production of acids by the body. The first of these, green food, also contains a number of alkaline substances for neutralizing acids.

GREEN FOOD

Green foods are preparations based on various green plants chosen specifically for their richness in vitamins, minerals, trace elements, and amino acids, as well as enzymes and chlorophyll. Developed to compensate for the deficiencies of the modern diet, which is poor in nutrients because of its refined nature and intensive factory-farm agricultural techniques, these products also help neutralize and eliminate acids.

As we have seen throughout this book, vegetables in general, but particularly green vegetables (salad greens, cabbage, broccoli, peppers, spinach, cucumbers, zucchini, etc.), are the principal and most generous source of alkaline minerals. This is why their consumption is recommended for the two main meals of the day, lunch and dinner. What we eat daily in the form of salads and raw and cooked vegetables generally covers the body's basic alkaline mineral needs, but this is far from sufficient to neutralize the many acids that have accumulated in the tissues of an acidified person. To neutralize these acids, the quantity of vegetables that would have to be consumed would not only be greater than anyone would be willing to eat, but it would also exceed their digestive capacity. There is a solution to this problem, however: vegetable juice.

Of course, juice lacks the fiber necessary for intestinal transit. But juices, just like green food, which is also prepared from a juice base, are supplements to, not substitutes for, a regular diet. The absence of fiber in juice concentrates the nutrients that were in the vegetables. Some of the plant's nutrients, including the alkaline minerals, are actually connected to the plant fiber. Even chewing thoroughly does not extract as much of these nutrients as do machines that pulverize the fiber to make juice. Separated from the framework of plant fiber, the nutrients are more available and easier to assimilate.

While the consumption of vegetable juice from broccoli, beets, spinach, and so on, or a blend of several, is quite beneficial, food supplements like green food use the plants richest in nutrients and alkaline minerals to supply the maximum possible active principles in the smallest possible volume. These plants are not those we usually eat, but the young sprouts of cereal grains, as well as those of forage plants used for livestock, such as wheat sprouts, barley grass, alfalfa sprouts, and kamut sprouts.

Wheat sprouts contain more alkaline minerals than any other sprouts or green vegetables: more than one hundred different nutrients, including almost all the minerals and trace elements, and the entire range of vitamins from the B group. The iron content of wheat sprouts, essential for good tissue oxygenation, is higher than that of spinach, which is considered to be one of the best sources for this mineral.

Wheat sprouts are the highest in chlorophyll of any plant source. Chlorophyll, which gives plants their green color, has a molecular structure that is almost identical to that of blood hemoglobin, which is indispensable for transporting oxygen into the cells. The similarity of chlorophyll to hemoglobin has led to the description of chlorophyll as the "blood" of the plant.

Chlorophyll plays an important role in deacidifying the body by oxygenating the tissues, enabling the tissues to oxidize many more weak and volatile acids than normal and eliminate them via respiration. But chlorophyll also has the property of breaking down carbon dioxide (which is acidic) and dissolving the deposits of strong acids, such as kidney stones. Furthermore, chlorophyll has diuretic and purifying properties that facilitate the elimination of acids.

Kamut is a very ancient wheat variety that has never been hybridized. Its grains are three times fatter than those of wheat, and their nutrient content, especially that of several alkaline minerals, is significantly higher. This richness is present in the juice of the young sprouts. Kamut juice is 90 percent higher in potassium, 148 percent higher in calcium, and 50 percent higher in iron than wheat juice; furthermore, the pH of this juice and the powder made from it is the most alkaline of all the green foods, which contributes to excellent deacidification of the body.

Barley grass has been recognized by researchers as the most nutritious plant in existence because of the number, variety, and concentration of the nutrients that go into its composition. Analyses of more than two hundred plants, algae, and herbs have shown that barley grass contains the most minerals, including a high concentration of alkaline minerals. Its vitamin B1 content (thiamine) is four times higher than that of wheat flour and thirty times higher than that of milk. Vitamin B1 is vital for the transformation and utilization of sugars, which, if not properly accomplished, leads to the production of numerous acids. Young barley grass is also the best natural source of the antioxidant superoxide dismutase (SOD), which prevents acidification of the tissues.

Alfalfa (also known as lucerne) is not a cereal grain like wheat, kamut, and barley but a legume like peanuts or soy. It is used as a forage plant for livestock

112

because of its high protein content, up to 55 percent of its total weight, and its high content of minerals such as calcium, iron, zinc, copper, and selenium, all alkaline minerals.

Commercially available green-food products vary in composition. Those most effective for deacidifying the body combine these four plants. Other legumes and plants, such as spirulina, may also be included, but these four plants should definitely be among them.

Because plant juices do not keep for long, green-food products are sold as either a powder of the sprouts themselves, a powder of the dried juice, or a combination of the two. Powder made from the juice is more concentrated and consequently more alkalizing than powder obtained from the ground leaves alone.

Green-food powder is available in capsules or as a powder to be mixed with water, making a drink with a distinctive but pleasant taste. Drinking it regularly every day provides the body with a host of alkaline minerals for deacidification purposes, but also with other nutrients, enzymes in particular, that fight against acidification indirectly by making metabolism more efficient and thus reducing the production of acids by the body.

ENZYME SUPPLEMENTS

People suffering from an acidified internal cellular environment are generally not eating enough vegetables, the principal food source for alkaline minerals. The result is a deficiency not only of alkaline substances, but also of enzymes. Enzymes play an important role for maintaining the acid–alkaline balance.

Enzymes are protein-based molecules that act as catalysts in biochemical reactions, triggering and supervising the reactions. Enzymes perform numerous transformations in the body without which it could not survive.

Every enzyme has a specific function that no other enzyme can perform. Enzymes are necessary for the digestion of proteins, fats, and carbohydrates and for their assimilation and incorporation into the tissues; for the production of energy; for cellular repair; for the breakdown and elimination of toxins; for the body's defense system; and so forth. There are thousands of enzymes in the body, acting in synergy. As each is responsible for only a specific part of the work, different enzymes work together, each stepping in at a specific moment and at a precise place in the long chain of biochemical transformations.

Enzymes are distributed throughout the cells and tissues, each type of enzyme located at the exact spot the body needs it. The body is constantly producing new enzymes to replace those that have been used. This production is not a quickand-easy process, though. It is sufficient to compensate for the normal loss of enzymes, but not when abnormal demands are made on the body at this level. Such demands are made in the digestion of cooked food.

Foods also contain enzymes, but they are very sensitive to heat. Too high a temperature during the cooking process destroys them. Cooked foods, whether boiled, steamed, or baked in an oven or microwave, are more or less impoverished of enzymes, depending on the mode of cooking used. Only the enzymes that survive the heat can take part in the digestion of the food from which they came. The body consequently has to supply the enzymes that were destroyed when the food was cooked; this gradually reduces its own reserves, especially if meals consist primarily or exclusively of cooked foods, if the individual overeats, or if the foods are refined (refined foods have already been stripped of a portion of their enzymes).

With these eating habits, which are followed by the majority of people today, over the long term the body's enzymatic capability shrinks. This means that biochemical transformations are not being performed as well, and that much more acid waste is produced during the metabolic process than normal. So just how does this occur?

As an illustration, let's take the transformation of glucose—that is, sugar—into energy. Because of the activity of various enzymes, glucose is first transformed into citric acid, then pyruvic acid, succinic acid, and fumaric acid in succession, ending finally as lactic acid. This acid is then attacked by another enzyme that transforms it into energy.

Normally, these transformations are carried out to the final stage, and the acids do not survive as acids because they have been converted into energy. But if there is an enzyme deficiency, the glucose transformation comes to a halt during the acid stages, and the result is acidification of the body's internal cellular environment, which would not occur if enough enzymes were available.

Transition through a series of acid stages also takes place when the body converts fats and proteins for its use. This process is so extensive that the inevitable consequence of any enzyme deficiency is acidification of the body. Of course, the more extensive the enzyme deficiency, the more acidic the body becomes, eventually resulting in illness. This process is exacerbated by the fact that an acid organic environment inhibits enzyme activity, thus reducing the enzymes' effectiveness and increasing the production of acid wastes even more.

To escape this vicious cycle, it is crucial to give the body the enzymes it needs. One way of doing this is to sharply increase consumption of raw vegetables at the two major meals of the day, noon and evening. Raw foods can be eaten either in the form of salad greens or as a side dish of colored vegetables like carrots or beets, or even as a mixed salad incorporating both. Thoroughly chewing these raw foods increases the benefit of this intake, because this frees more enzymes from the cellulose framework that binds them.

The benefits offered by a larger intake of enzymes can be easily seen: a cooked meal is digested more easily when raw foods have been added to it. We feel lighter after a meal accompanied by salad or raw vegetables because the digestion of the enzyme-poor cooked foods has been facilitated by the extra enzymes contributed by the raw foods.

Another way for the body to obtain the enzymes it needs is via enzymatic supplements. This additional support is often essential, because eating more raw foods is sufficient to address only minor enzyme deficiencies and maintain the proper acid–alkaline balance; if an individual's enzymatic capacity has been overdrawn, deacidification requires a contribution of enzymes from supplements in addition to those supplied by the food in the diet.

To be effective, these supplements should contain a wide variety of enzymes to respond to the body's many needs:

- bromelain, papain, trypsin, etc., to digest proteins
- lipase, etc., to digest fats
- amylase, malt diastase, invertase, etc., to digest carbohydrates
- cellulase and hemicullulase to break down fruit and vegetable fiber
- serrazimes to digest wastes and dead cells

The enzymes in commercial supplements are prepared so that they retain their properties even after they have entered the digestive tract, resisting stomach acids and other substances that could destroy them on their way to the cells. Taken on a daily basis in combination with a diet high in raw vegetables, the enzymes supplied by supplements should cause a sharp reduction in the body's level of acidification. They help the body burn acids away, contributing to a quicker restoration of the body's pH.

PREBIOTICS AND PROBIOTICS

The intestines are home to several hundred billion microorganisms belonging to more than four hundred different species. All together, these microorganisms are known as the *intestinal flora.*

The presence of these microorganisms in the intestines is necessary for the body to function. They play a role in the digestion of foods, facilitate the assimilation of nutrients, stimulate intestinal transit, produce vitamins B and K, and neutralize poisons. Simply by their presence, they also prevent harmful microorganisms from multiplying.

Under normal circumstances, the four hundred to five hundred varieties of microorganisms that make up the healthy intestinal flora cohabit harmoniously. A balance is maintained between the sizes of these different populations, the areas of the territories they occupy, the sections of the intestines they colonize, and the portions of the foods to which each has a right.

Because they are so precisely distributed, it is very difficult for foreign microorganisms to invade in force; all the niches in the intestines for microorganisms to reside and thrive are already being judiciously exploited. The

115

intestines are, in fact, the natural living environment for the intestinal flora, so none of them are prepared to surrender their place to invaders. They fight against invasion by secreting antibiotic substances that kill the invaders, and by vigorously occupying and defending their terrain.

In addition to a large number of harmless and beneficial microorganisms that fall under the general heading of probiotics (*pro* means "for"; *bio* means "life"), the intestinal flora also harbors various pathogens (microorganisms that can cause disease), which play a distinct role in the digestive process. Normally their dangerous nature cannot manifest because of their limited numbers, and they remain in the minority as long as the intestinal flora is healthy.

But when the intestinal flora has been weakened or partially decimated— which can occur when the diet includes too much meat, refined foods, and chemical additives; when a person is stressed; or when the individual has taken too many antibiotics—it becomes incapable of acting as a protective barrier, and it will allow some pathogens to multiply and trigger an infection.

Candida albicans, for example, is a normal resident of the intestines. Usually its population is quite limited, and it plays an insignificant role. It would probably have remained completely unknown to the general public if the destruction of the intestinal flora by antibiotic abuse had not allowed it to expand its growth excessively in large numbers of people. When this occurs, *C. albicans* colonizes the digestive tract, where it creates a number of different disorders (gas, bloating, colitis, etc.), as well spreading into other parts of the body. It is implicated in a large number of fungal diseases (mycoses) as well as certain nervous disorders.

In addition to *C. albicans,* other yeasts and fungi, all categorized under the generic term of microforms, can increase in number to the extent that they partially replace the normal intestinal flora. Like all living creatures, these microforms secrete acidic wastes. These can include, for example, oxalic acid, lactic acid, and citric acid. When the number of microforms that release these wastes are limited, it is of no great consequence. Among a large number of people, however, because of the imbalance of their intestinal flora, the population of such pathogens increases substantially to proportions that are higher than they should be. There are thus many more microforms that secrete acids and consequently all that many more acids to threaten the acid–alkaline balance of the body.

The initial proliferation of these microforms sets up a vicious circle: by acidifying the internal cellular environment with their wastes, they create an environment that is favorable for them. The more they acidify their environment, the more they are able to multiply. The increase of their population then engenders an increased production of acid toxins that acidify the body even further.

Too great a number of these microforms acidifies the body in yet other ways. On one hand, they force the body to give up numerous alkaline substances to neutralize their acids, increasing the acidification of the cellular environment; on the other hand, a portion of the alkaline substances that are carried into the body

116

by foods is eaten by these microforms, making it unavailable for the body's own fight against acidification. Furthermore, too great a presence of microforms—and consequently too weak a presence of probiotic microorganisms—hampers digestion. The fermentation caused by incomplete digestion produces numerous acids that combine with the others, increasing the body's acidification.

How can we combat the acidification resulting from excessive colonization by microforms?

There are two methods available for remedying this situation: we can take prebiotics and probiotics. Both strengthen and increase the number of beneficial intestinal flora, reducing the living space available to microforms and thus cutting down the size of their populations.

Prebiotics are foods or substances that constitute a food of choice for beneficial microorganisms. Providing them with optimal nourishment makes them stronger and enables them to multiply more easily. When prebiotics are provided to microorganisms in abundance, their populations can grow larger, because easily available food ensures the nutritional needs of a larger population.

Prebiotics are the fibers found in foods of plant origin: vegetables, fruits, cereals, and beans. Human digestive juices cannot break these fibers down, but the beneficial microorganisms of the intestines can. Among these prebiotics are inulin and fructo-oligosaccharide (FOS), which, as carbohydrates, serve plants as an energy reserve. They can be found, for example, in onions, asparagus, artichokes, chicory roots, and leeks.

The regular consumption of inulin enables the intestines' population of beneficial microorganisms to multiply ten times. Inulin has the property as well of encouraging the absorption of calcium by the body, which helps in deacidification, since calcium is an alkaline mineral.

When you become acidified and your intestinal flora is out of balance—which is revealed by poor digestion—it is essential that you supply the remaining intestinal microorganisms with the prebiotics they need so badly. You can do this by increasing your consumption of salad greens and both raw and cooked vegetables, as well as other plant-based foods, but also by taking prebiotic complexes that are specially manufactured to ensure optimal nutrition. Concentrated and easily assimilated by the beneficial microorganisms of the intestinal flora, the prebiotics encourage them to multiply.

Certain prebiotic complexes contain, in addition to FOS and inulin, soy fiber and fiber from other plants. The best-known property of these fibers is to encourage intestinal transit, but they can also hold onto the wastes in the intestines, including acid wastes, so that they are not absorbed by the body but carried out with the stools, which diminishes the body's acidification.

The second means of fighting the proliferation of microforms is to take probiotics. Probiotics are used mainly when the intestinal flora has been sharply reduced. In this situation, it is not enough to provide the remaining microorganisms with proper nutrition. The competition with the microforms is too brutal for the beneficial microorganisms to multiply rapidly, so more radical methods are called for. This method consists of bringing into the intestines a large number of microorganisms from the outside by eating foods like probiotic yogurt, which contain a very high number of these microorganisms.

To obtain a more substantial intake of probiotic microorganisms than that available from yogurt, and consequently to restore the intestinal flora more efficiently and quickly, there are several products made from lyophilized microorganisms. Lyophilization involves the delicate freeze-drying of microorganisms without killing them. They are then placed in capsules that protect them from the digestive juices of the stomach. Each capsule can contain from tens of millions of these microorganisms to as many as several billion. When the capsule reaches the warm, moist environment of the intestine, it dissolves, and the germs rehydrate and emerge from their imposed sleep. Once they have become active again, they colonize the intestines and start to multiply there, which they can do even more easily if they are supplied with all the prebiotics they require for food. This is why it is often recommended to take prebiotic and probiotic complexes simultaneously. The microorganisms most often used for these products are *Lactobacillus acidophilus, L. rhamnosus,* and *L. casei,* as well as *Bifidobacterium bifidum* and *B. longdum,* to name but a few.

An upsurge of microforms that produce acid toxins is a little-known factor in the acidification of the body, but it is of major importance for individuals who are suffering from an imbalance in their intestinal flora, candidiasis, or other fungal infections.

ANTIOXIDANTS

Antioxidants are substances that neutralize the harmful and partially acidifying activity of free radicals. But just what are free radicals, and how do they contribute to the acidification of the body?

Isolated atoms can have either an even or odd number of electrons (the small electrical charges that revolve around the nucleus), but when they combine with other atoms to form molecules, the molecules always have an even number of electrons. There is only one exception: free radicals. These are chemical units that, instead of having an even number of electrons as is the rule, have an odd number. The odd number of electrons makes free radicals highly unstable and therefore reactive, because the solitary electron is making every effort to find another electron with which it can bond in order to stabilize.

This quest is nonselective; the free radical attacks any molecule with which it comes into contact in order to steal an electron. But when it steals this electron, it transforms the other molecule into a free radical, as the latter now has an odd number of electrons.

The theft of an electron is not innocuous for a molecule, because it alters or destroys its structure. Free-radical activity is therefore always destructive. If this molecule is part of a cell, the cell is stricken or destroyed. When, for example, a cell membrane is broken by a free radical, the cell loses its contents and dies. When its DNA is struck, it can no longer multiply; when its mitochondria are affected, it can no longer breathe; and so forth. Useful substances like enzymes, red corpuscles, and vitamins can also be destroyed. The destructive capabilities of free radicals are used by the body itself. The immune system, for example, intentionally creates a certain number of free radicals to destroy microbes or their toxins.

The lifespan of free radicals is quite short, from one to ten millionths of a second. The body's normal functioning creates free radicals. But added to this physiological production of free radicals are those brought into the body by denatured and spoiled foods, tobacco smoke, pollution, radioactivity, and so on. External sources of free radicals are quite numerous.

The harmful activity of free radicals is not the primary cause of acidification, but it makes a contribution. The destruction of cells, DNA, proteins, and various other useful substances creates acid wastes, such as uric acid, phosphoric acid, and sulfuric acid. Of course, the body has to deal with the death of some of its cells and the exhaustion of its tissues on a daily basis. But the acids resulting from the destruction caused by free radicals adds to the body's normal acid production.

Furthermore, the free radicals' damage to and destruction of cells forces the body to react to neutralize and repair the damage, intensify cellular multiplication, and produce new enzymes and proteins. The increased metabolic activity this requires is stressful to the body—and any prolonged stress has an acidifying effect.

Fortunately, the body does not lack defenses against free radicals. It can produce substances called antioxidants that neutralize free radicals by supplying them with the electron they are missing.

Why are these substances called antioxidants? Free radicals are actually an oxygen derivative, and their destructiveness is the result of oxidizing the substances with which they come in contact, causing a kind of burn. Antioxidants, as the name suggests, prevent this from taking place.

Several vitamins have an antioxidant effect, such as vitamins A, E, C, the flavonoids (vitamin P), and certain trace elements like selenium and zinc. But there are plants that contain even more potent antioxidants. The antioxidant proanthocyanidin (OPC), for example, which is forty times stronger than flavonoids, can be found in grape seeds and in various small fruits (blackberries, bilberries, cranberries, strawberries, blueberries, and so on); the catechin extracted from green tea is 200 times stronger than vitamin E; and the proanthocyanidin extract from pine bark is fifty times stronger than vitamin E and twenty times stronger than vitamin C.

There are several antioxidant complexes available on the market manufactured from extracts of these substances. These are provided as complexes because different kinds of antioxidants are needed to address the

119

different kinds of free radicals. The concentration of these complexes is such that one capsule per day supplies enough antioxidants to cover the body's basic needs.

9

Draining Acids

Up to now, the main topic of this book has been how to reduce the accumulation of acids through adequate diet and alkaline supplements.

However, there are two causes for acidification of the body's internal environment. One is the ingestion of excessive amounts of acids; the other is their insufficient elimination. This chapter examines how to stimulate the organs responsible for elimination so they can get rid of as much acid as possible.

The organs responsible for the elimination of acids are the kidneys and skin, on the one hand, and the lungs on the other. It is important to make a distinction between these two groups of organs of elimination, because they each deal with different kinds of acids. The skin and kidneys eliminate strong acids, such as uric acid, sulfuric acid, and phosphoric acid—the acids that primarily come from animal proteins. The lungs eliminate the weak or volatile acids, such as citric acid, pyruvic acid, oxalic acid, and so forth, that derive from plants in the form of carbon dioxide (CO_2).

ACID DRAINAGE THROUGH THE KIDNEYS

Although they can eliminate weak acids, the kidneys specialize in the treatment of strong acids. This elimination is limited in quantity, because it is a relatively difficult task requiring a complex set of procedures. First the wastes have to be filtered out of the blood. Next they are diluted in fluid so they do not cause injury to the mucous membranes of the urinary system. They are then conducted to the bladder, where they are stored until they are expelled from the body by urination.

The quantity of acids that the kidneys eliminate each day may not match the quantity of acids consumed and produced by the body on that day. Dietary reform that reduces the intake of acids helps, but it is also important to stimulate the kidneys to increase the amounts of acids they filter and void, especially for people whose kidneys operate below their actual capacity. This is not a matter of kidney disease but rather of an insufficiency or renal laziness.

A primary means of stimulating the work of the kidneys is to increase the amount of liquids you consume. A major aspect of the renal filtration process is the difference between the blood pressure that pushes into the renal filter and the opposing resistance of this filter. If the blood pressure is greater than that of the filter, the blood is pushed through the filter and its acids removed. In the opposite case, the filtration works poorly because the lack of pressure is a hindrance. By drinking more than usual you can increase your blood volume, which then exerts greater pressure. The inevitable result is more copious urination.

The role played by pressure in urination explains why coffee—which raises blood pressure—increases urination, and also why fear stimulates the need to urinate (adrenaline secretion raises blood pressure).

An effective way of drinking enough liquid over the course of the day—and an easy way to remember to do so—is to systematically have a drink after each time you urinate. Urination is prompted by an amount of liquid in the body over a certain tolerance threshold. Voiding this liquid through urination reduces the amount of liquid until it is beneath the threshold of tolerance, and it remains below this threshold as long as no new liquid has been drunk. Taking a drink immediately following urination, in a quantity equal to or greater than what was eliminated, causes the liquid level of the body to rise above the tolerance threshold again, and this triggers a new elimination cycle automatically.

The volume of liquid that thus travels through the body encourages the elimination of toxins, because it can easily dilute and transport numerous acids and salts without causing the urine to become overly concentrated. The bed of a stream is much cleaner if large quantities of water flow through it as opposed to a small sluggish current.

Medicinal Plants for Draining Acids

While an abundant supply of liquid encourages elimination, it is also possible to increase the quantity of acids eliminated from the body by stimulating the kidneys' filtration capacities with diuretic (urination-producing) medicinal plants. These plants and herbs allow the kidneys to handle much larger quantities of toxins, and the body is therefore able to get rid of those toxins much more quickly.

Through the action of these plants the renal filter first gets rid of the wastes that are burdening it. Once this has been accomplished, it cleanses the blood of any acids it is holding, allowing those just outside the blood capillaries—the acids embedded a little deeper in the tissues—to enter the circulatory system and be transported to the kidneys. Once these acids have been eliminated, those embedded even deeper in the tissues enter the circulatory system for eventual removal. Such an elimination process reaches progressively deeper tissues until, finally, the body's entire internal environment is cleansed.

To be really effective, diuretic plants must be taken in the proper dosages; people usually do not take enough, and so have minimal or no results. With the correct dosages the effects are unmistakable. As the urine becomes more heavily charged with acids it takes on a darker color, and the odor becomes stronger. The frequency of urination increases, as does the quantity of urine eliminated.

To determine the optimum dosage, you need to increase the average doses suggested until you obtain the desired effects. Diuretic plant medicines should be taken three times daily at least—morning, noon, and in the evening before supper. This ensures that the kidneys can depend on their support for the entire day. These therapies should last anywhere from four to six weeks and be renewed after a break of a week or two for a total of two to three rounds. It is also a good idea to vary the plants used from one therapeutic session to another, as the body has a tendency to become accustomed to any given plant and stops reacting as strongly to the stimulus the plant provides after a certain period.

As with foods, some of these plants (primarily horsetail—rich in silicic acid—and birch) also contain acids and thus should not be taken by people with metabolic-acid deficiencies.

When prepared as teas, diuretic plants enter the body in liquid form, thus intensifying their effect. However, preparing them this way does take a little time, and not everyone enjoys drinking these teas. Fortunately most plants are also available in tablet form and as tinctures, both equally valid alternatives. These forms are also more practical for when you are traveling or eating out at a restaurant. The list below defines the various means of preparing plant medicines.

PLANT MEDICINE PREPARATIONS

Tea or infusion: A drink obtained by steeping a plant or herb in hot water for several minutes.

Decoction: A beverage obtained by boiling plant material in water in a tightly sealed pot.

Tinctures (drops): A solution of a plant's active principles in an alcohol base.

Tablets: Medicinal plants are dried, crushed into a powder, and compacted into tablet form.

Tisane: A mixture of different plants prepared as a tea.

Many plants are available to assist the kidneys in draining acids from the body. The list below gives several recommendations for plant therapies and the best methods of preparation. In these recipes a "cup" refers to the standard six-ounce teacup.

PLANT MEDICINES FOR KIDNEY STIMULATION

- Black currant: The leaves have a diuretic quality and make a very pleasant-tasting beverage. Make a tea by mixing 1 handful of leaves (1^1/2 oz; 40 g) per quart of water, or 1 tablespoon per cup. Steep at least 10 minutes. Drink 3 cups daily before or between meals.

- Artichoke: The leaves (not the bracts of the flowers) have an excellent diuretic effect. They also stimulate liver function. Artichoke leaves make a bitter-tasting drink. Mix 1/3 oz (10 g) of leaves per quart of water, or 1 teaspoonful per cup. Steep for 10 minutes. Drink 3 cups a day before meals.

- Cherry stems: The peduncles, or stems, are used for their diuretic action. Save the stems when you eat cherries and put them aside to dry. This makes a very refreshing beverage. Mix 1 handful of stems per quart of water. Make a decoction by boiling for 10 minutes. Drink 3 cups a day at a minimum.

- Linden bark: Linden bark is an excellent means for draining acids from the body (also recommended for all forms of rheumatism, kidney stones, and gallstones). Make a decoction by mixing 1 1/2 oz (40 g) of bark per quart of water. Boil until the liquid is reduced to 1/4 of the volume. Drink the decoction during the day. Traditional therapy calls for this beverage to be drunk 20 days a month for several months.

- Pilosella: An excellent diuretic and disinfectant for the urinary tract. Take 30–50 drops of pilosella tincture in a little water 3 times a day before meals.

- Cranberry: Cranberry is a diuretic well known for its disinfectant effect on the urinary tract. Take 20–40 drops with a little water 3 times a day before meals. (Cranberry juice is also an effective diuretic and anti-infective.)

- Couch grass: Couch grass is an excellent cleansing plant. Its preferred use is in tablet form because of its flavor. Take 1–3 tablets with a little water 3 times a day just before meals.

- Ash: A good eliminator of acids, ash, when taken in large doses, has a purgative effect. Take 1–3 tablets with a little water 3 times a day just before meals.

Some additional plant medicines and methods of preparation include:

- Goldenrod, ash, and parietaria (pellitory): For each plant mix 1–2 tablespoons per cup of water. Steep for 10 minutes. Drink 3 cups daily.

- Black currant, corn silk, couch grass, elder, licorice, orthosiphon (cat's whisker), thistle: For each plant mix 1–2 tablespoons per cup of water. Boil for 2 minutes, then steep 10 minutes. Drink 3 cups daily.

There are numerous commercial blends of diuretic plants available as tisanes, tinctures, tablets, and so on. These preparations are generally very effective and provide great benefit to the user.

Whey Treatment for Draining Acids

Whey is the liquid obtained from the coagulation of milk. It is released when curds are strained. The detoxifying qualities of whey have been known since antiquity. Its diuretic properties are what interest us here.

Whey owes its powerful diuretic effect to its high potassium content. By forcing excess salt out of the body, potassium prompts the elimination of fluids retained because of the presence of sodium—fluids that contain, among other things, acids. The large quantities of whey that are ingested during the course of this treatment—up to 2 to 3 quarts a day—cause the kidneys to work more intensively. The great English doctor Thomas Sydenham (1624–89) specifically—and successfully—recommended whey as a treatment for gout, an illness caused by excess acid, particularly uric acid.

The benefits of whey for restoring the body's optimum acid–alkaline balance go beyond its ability to stimulate elimination. It is also rich in minerals (around 5 percent of its dried weight), primarily alkaline minerals such as potassium, calcium, and magnesium, which all contribute to addressing alkaline deficiencies.

Whey's alkalizing property is effective only when the whey is fresh, because whey acidifies very quickly. Even a few hours following its manufacture, whey can lose its alkaline properties. This was a very common problem in the past when treatments used only liquid whey. Today whey is available in powdered form; the powdering process arrests acidification. Sold in health food stores, it is also flavored with natural fruit extracts. The whey is reconstituted by mixing it with water according to the manufacturer's instructions. Once it has been reconstituted the liquid should be drunk quickly (within an hour), before it becomes acidic.

During the treatment, drink from three to five glasses to 2 to 3 pints of whey a day.

It is necessary, however, to give the body time to adapt. On the first day of the treatment drink only one eight-ounce glass of whey; on the second day, two glasses; and so on until you reach five glasses per day. That amount is maintained for the remainder of the treatment, which normally lasts between two and three weeks. (For those who are interested, I have written extensively on this therapy in my *La cure de petit-lait,* Geneva: Editions Jouvence, 1994.)

ACID DRAINAGE THROUGH THE SKIN

Just like the kidneys, the sweat glands allow strong acids to be removed from the body. There are between 140 and 240 of these glands per square inch of skin, which adds up to around two million of these glands in the body.

The sweat glands filter out acids and toxins carried by the blood, sending them toward the body's surface, diluted in water (sweat). The blood that carries these waste products circulates in extremely fine vessels, the capillaries. Consequently, perspiration can only be abundant if there is good subcutaneous blood circulation. This can be encouraged by physical exercise, saunas, and hot baths. The muscular contractions of physical activity stimulate blood circulation, while heat causes the capillaries to dilate and also accelerates the speed with which the blood circulates.

Under normal circumstances the skin secretes between one and one and a half quarts of sweat a day. We are normally not aware of this, as the sweat evaporates immediately. Sedentary people may sweat as little as a pint a day. Elimination of acids through the skin in this case is minimal.

When stimulated by intense exercise, the skin can eliminate a pint of sweat in one hour, and considerably more if the exercise is followed by a sauna. An hour in a sauna can discharge one to one and a half quarts of sweat.

An individual suffering from a high fever eliminates similar quantities, if not more, of sweat.

Hyperthermal Baths

Insufficient elimination of acids through the skin can be corrected by physical exercise and saunas. A less well-known method is hot baths, or hyperthermal therapy. All that is required is a bathtub and hot water. The heat causes an artificial fever, which in turn stimulates a large amount of perspiration, and therefore a significant elimination of acids. Hyperthermal baths have a retraining effect on the skin. If you have poor perspiration you will, as a rule, perspire more freely after several baths.

Get into the bath when the water is at a temperature of 98.6° Fahrenheit (37° Celsius), or body tempeature, then raise the water temperature gradually by adding hot water just up to your comfort threshold. Do not bring the water to the hottest temperature you can endure; it should not be so hot that you are uncomfortable. You should be able to remain in the bath for a good quarter hour. Depending on your tolerance for heat, the temperature of the bath will be between 102° and 108° Fahrenheit (between 39° and 42° Celsius), or sometimes higher.

The purpose of this hyperthermal bath is to envelop the body in high heat. If you cannot tolerate high temperatures at all, you can still benefit by spending a longer time in the tub with the water at a comfortable temperature.

It is crucial that you allow the body to get used to the hot baths gradually, increasing the temperature and lengthening the time spent in the tub in small increments over a period of several weeks before reaching your comfort limits.

It is not advisable to get right into a steaming-hot bath even after you have built up a good tolerance. When confronted by this sudden thermal assault, the body's defenses close the pores of the skin. They are then very slow to reopen, sabotaging the purpose of the bath. So warm the bath up slowly after you get in.

When the bath is done, wrap yourself in a towel and a blanket and rest for half an hour to allow the body to finish perspiring and recover its equilibrium.

Depending on your level of vitality you can take such a bath every day for a period of two to three weeks, or every other day for several months. It is best to schedule the bath for the evening hours because it relaxes the body and encourages sound sleep.

When the body is bathed in hot water, its own internal temperature rapidly increases. This can be easily verified by taking a reading with an oral thermometer. As stated earlier, the hyperthermal bath creates an artificial fever that has the same characteristics as a genuine, natural fever.

Fever is a means of defense the body uses during illness to intensify the metabolic process and accelerate the burning-off of waste products—acids among others—that saturate the body's internal environment, as well as to make that environment inhospitable to the survival and reproduction of pathogens (bacteria and viruses). It is therefore a beneficial reaction that allows the body to rapidly bring its condition back to normal.

When the combustion of waste products is intensified during a fever, they are degraded and distributed throughout the body to furnish fuel for energy or cell-building material. This includes combustion of the noncirculating toxins that are deeply embedded in the body's tissues.

If you implement hyperthermal therapy too quickly you can unleash a massive discharge of deeply embedded toxins, causing what is known as a cleansing crisis. When the embedded toxins are brought suddenly to the circulatory level and added to the toxins already in circulation, the ability of the organs of elimination to oxidize and get rid of them can easily be overwhelmed. Some very unpleasant symptoms, such as headaches, nausea, and rheumatic-like crises, can result. These can be avoided by starting the therapy gradually and by draining the acids in circulation before starting an intensive hyperthermal treatment.

Drinking a sweat-stimulating tisane before and after the bath is also useful. During the bath, the skin's eliminatory work can be enhanced by scrubbing or massage.

Using Medicinal Plants for Eliminating Acids through the Skin

Medicinal plants that increase the secretion of sweat can also increase the quantity of acids eliminated from the body. Usually, however, the increased perspiration is noticeable only when the body has a reason to sweat, such as in the case of heat or physical exertion. Nevertheless, by regularly taking sweat-stimulating substances you can help your clogged pores clean themselves and work more actively.

These preparations should be taken three times daily, and the infusions should be well heated. The effect of hyperthermal baths, sweating sessions in the sauna, and physical exercise is reinforced by drinking one to two piping hot cups of a tea brewed from sweat-stimulating herbs before and after a session.

Here are several examples of medicinal plants that have sweat-stimulating properties.

MEDICINAL PLANTS FOR ELIMINATING ACIDS THROUGH THE SKIN

- Elder: The flowers of the elder are sweat-stimulating and diuretic, and they make a very pleasant and flavorful drink. Mix 1 tablespoon of flowers per cup of hot water as an infusion. Steep for 10 minutes. Drink 3 cups daily.

- Linden: A highly popular plant, linden has long been used for its sweat-stimulating and sedative properties. Prepare as an infusion by mixing 1 heaping handful of flowers per cup of hot water, or $1/2$ to 1 oz (15–30 g) per quart. Steep for 10 minutes. Drink 3 or more cups daily.

- Burdock: This plant, a diuretic, promotes bile production; it is also a laxative. Burdock is often recommended as a treatment for skin disorders. Prepare as a decoction by mixing $1 1/2$ oz (40 g) of root per quart of water. Boil for 10 minutes. Drink 3 or more cups per day. Or take 40 drops with water 3 times a day before meals.

- Wild pansy: This plant is very effective in treating skin disorders. In addition to its sweat-stimulating qualities, it is a good overall purifier. Take 20–50 drops with water 3 times a day before meals.

Plant medicines can also be prepared as tisanes and used for stimulating sweat. Linden, elder flowers, borage, balm, violet, meadowsweet, wild pansy, chamomile, sloe flowers, and primrose are all good for use as tisanes. Mix 1 tablespoon of plant matter per cup. Steep for 10 minutes. Drink 3 cups per day.

ACID DRAINAGE THROUGH THE LUNGS

The lungs play a dual role in the elimination of acid wastes from the body. On the one hand, they supply the tissues with oxygen so volatile acids can be oxidized. It is not enough for oxygen to fill the respiratory tract; the oxygen must be conducted into the tissues by the bloodstream so that the oxidation of acid wastes can occur there. On the other hand, acids are rejected by the respiratory tract in the form of carbon dioxide (CO_2). Produced within the tissues (and present there in liquid form), this carbon dioxide must make its way to the lungs and be expelled in sufficient quantity that the body is truly rid of it.

Since everyone breathes, you might wonder why there should be any problem eliminating acid wastes through the respiratory tract. But not everyone breathes the same way; breathing rate and air flow can vary significantly from one person to another, and in the same person at different times. A person at rest takes in a pint of air per breath, whereas an active individual takes in twice that much. At the height of a game an athlete may inhale 5 to 6 quarts every breath, ten to twelve times as much as a person at rest.

Although a pint of breath is enough for an individual at rest or asleep, it is insufficient for even a sedentary person working and eating. The greater the rate of activity or amount of food eaten, the greater need the body has of oxygen. When the body does not get enough oxygen to meet its needs, oxidation is poor, and this increases the accumulation of acids. Furthermore, as the volume of air exhaled is reduced, so is the quantity of carbon dioxide that is eliminated. The result is acidification of the body by weak acids.

Of course, acidification of the body is even greater when a person smokes. Tobacco smoking not only reduces the intake of oxygen, and therefore the oxidation of acids in the tissues, but by hardening the lungs it diminishes the elimination of carbon dioxide. Furthermore, by constantly stimulating the nervous system, tobacco creates a state of stress in the body, resulting in the production of many acids. The more acidified the body becomes by smoking, the more tired the smoker is and the greater is his or her urge to smoke again. Because it lowers a person's need to smoke, alkalizing the inner environment is one of the best means of enabling a smoker to kick the habit.

A properly functioning oxidation system has beneficial effects on the body's pH. If you work seated in a poorly ventilated office for an entire afternoon you are prone to acidification. If you were to measure your urinary pH at that time it would be around 5 or 6. After you took a brisk walk outside in the fresh air, however, the pH would climb back up to 7 without your having to eat any alkaline food or take an alkaline supplement. But this is only true when the cause of acidification is a lack of oxygen.

Physical activity stimulates larger inhalations and exhalations, so any aerobic exercise (walking, jogging, riding a bicycle, gymnastics, and so on) is a great help in draining acids. Daily exercise is most effective because it facilitates the oxidation and elimination of volatile acids as they are produced. Accordingly, it is preferable to walk every day for thirty minutes in the fresh air than to take a three-hour walk on the weekend.

It is clear to see that the elimination of weak acids is much easier than that of strong acids; the latter can only be voided by the kidneys in fixed daily amounts. There is, however, no set daily limit for the elimination of weak (volatile) acid wastes, which are eliminated in proportion to the oxygenation that occurs during the day.

INTESTINAL DRAINAGE

As we have already seen, a number of intestinal microorganisms produce acid wastes. These are primarily fungi, yeasts, and molds (or microforms) that live in the intestines and form part of the intestinal flora.

Like all living organisms, these microforms excrete wastes created by the metabolism of their food. These wastes are varied and high in number. *Candida albicans,* for example, secretes several hundred different kinds of wastes (mycotoxins), some of which are acid. All the microforms together excrete more than a thousand different toxins.

Microforms are commensal microbes; that is, they are legitimate residents of the body. They require glucose as an energetic fuel and fat and proteins to develop and grow. To obtain these nutrients, they break down substances in the alimentary bolus (a mass of chewed food in the stomach) into particles small enough for them to use, thus playing a role in the digestive process.

As long as the number of microforms inhabiting the intestines is small, their presence is beneficial; but when they multiply out of control, they cause health problems. Overpopulation of the intestines by microforms creates indigestion, heartburn, cramps, diarrhea, and other complaints. When the space available in the intestinal environment becomes too small for the microform populations to expand, some of them leave and colonize other areas of the body. For example, when they set up shop in the mouth, they cause thrush; on the skin in the corners of the mouth, perleche; in the lungs, respiratory problems; and in the bladder, cystitis.

Why do microforms sometimes breed to such excess in the intestines? An inadequate diet is one reason, as it encourages the proliferation of microforms at the expense of the other microorganisms in the intestinal flora. Repeated use of antibiotics produces the same result. Chronically bad digestion also alters the intestinal environment—and thus the living conditions of the microforms— because of the constant fermentation created by poorly digested food. Constipation is also a cause because the wastes, instead of being rapidly eliminated from the body, accumulate internally. In all these cases, the intestinal environment becomes favorable for microforms and allows them to multiply.

Microforms love being inside an intestine full of food and wastes. In fact, the more the quality of the intestinal environment deteriorates, the more favorable it becomes for them. This kind of environment is acid and allows them to multiply easily. But because the wastes these microforms eliminate are also acidic, the more they multiply, the more they acidify the intestine, making it even more favorable for their survival and multiplication.

The acids created by microform overgrowth do not remain in the intestines. They are absorbed by the walls of the intestines and enter the bloodstream. From there they are reallocated to all parts of the body, where they join the acids in the tissues that have been created at the cellular level.

To bring a halt to this common cause of acidification and clear up fungal diseases and chronic candidiasis, it is imperative to cleanse the intestines. Only by ridding the intestines of the wastes and surplus microforms can this kind of acid production be halted and a long-lasting deacidification process take hold. Otherwise, the acids that have been successfully neutralized and eliminated by changing to a healthier diet and taking supplements are constantly replaced by new acids produced by these microforms.

The intestines can be cleansed by either mechanical or chemical means. Substances that cleanse the intestines mechanically stimulate peristalsis by their volume, weight, and consistency. The plant fiber contained in fruits, vegetables, and whole grains, as well as in seeds like flax that are especially high in fiber, fills the intestines and brushes the nerve endings in the intestinal wall, triggering reflex contraction of the intestines, which pushes the contents toward the exit. Flax seeds also contain mucilage and oils that lubricate the intestines and help the contents slide through more easily.

Drinking large volumes of water—3 to 4 liters a day—also stimulates the intestines by filling them, dissolving their contents, and exerting pressure on the intestinal walls, which react by increasing their peristaltic movement. Water can also be introduced into the colon by enemas. Here too, the pressure of the water encourages the elimination of wastes.

The chemicals used to stimulate the intestines come from medicinal plants, which contain special substances that trigger and activate peristaltic activity by acting on the nerves and muscles of the intestines. This causes the contents of the intestines to be pushed farther down and toward the exit.

A large variety of plants can be used for this purpose: dried alder buckthorn bark, senna, mallow, barberry, cascara sagrada, goldenseal, and others. (Note that buckthorn bark is toxic to the body when fresh—the medicinal form of the plant has been dried for over a year.) Some examples of plant preparations follow.

- Alder buckthorn: This is a gentle laxative. The bark of this tree stimulates the intestines without irritating them, making it suitable for everyone. It also has an effect on the liver. Three times a day before meals, take 15–30 drops of alder buckthorn tincture, mixed with a little water.

- Mallow: The leaves and flowers of the mallow plant also have a gentle and nonirritating laxative effect on the intestines. Preparations made from this plant are often recommended for chronic constipation, especially when the digestive tract is inflamed. Take 20–50 drops of mallow tincture, blended with a little water, three times a day before meals. For an infusion, steep a handful of dried leaves and flowers for 10 minutes in water that has previously been brought to a boil. Drink a cup of this infusion before each meal.

There are a large number of plants with laxative properties. The commercial blends for intestinal cleansing generally contain several plants, including those mentioned above and others. Because the active properties of such blended preparations are more numerous and varied than those of a single plant, their action is more reliable and complete, as they stimulate the intestines in a number of different ways.

To increase the efficiency of these blends, betonite clay is sometimes added. The clay is not itself a laxative, but it has the unusual property of attracting and holding toxins, acids, and pathogens like the microforms that stagnate in the intestines. Laden with acids and microforms, the clay then leaves the intestines mixed into the stools. As betonite clay can sometimes have a dehydrating effect on the stools, it is good to drink a lot of liquids when using it.

Proper intestinal functioning depends on good bile production by the liver, as the bile stimulates peristaltic activity and lubricates the intestines. It is recommended to use liver-supporting plants at the same time as laxative plants. Some possibilities follow.

- Milk thistle: The leaves of this plant provide excellent support to the work of the liver. They also possess an overall tonic effect. As a tincture, take 20–40 drops mixed with water 3 times a day before meals. The tea is prepared by dropping a handful of leaves to steep for ten minutes in water that has been previously brought to a boil. Drink 3 cups a day.

- Boldo: The leaves of this Chilean tree encourage bile secretion. Drink 3 cups a day of an infusion of 1 teaspoon of leaves steeped in boiled water for 10 minutes. As a tincture, take 30–50 drops blended with water 3 times a day before meals.

Other hepatic plants may also be used—angelica, Japanese wasabi, rosemary, dandelion, and so on. These plants and others like them can be found in commercially available blends for the liver. They are sometimes combined with sulfur and specific amino acids (N-acetyl cysteine, L-taurine) as well as with grapefruit-seed extract and olive-leaf extract; these substances can destroy the fungi, yeasts, and molds living in the intestines.

To cleanse the intestines thoroughly, a purification treatment should be followed for a minimum of two to three days, but it is preferable to extend it over a period of two to three weeks. To get rid of the wastes and microforms that have been accumulating in the intestines for months, if not longer, the intestines should be stimulated regularly several times a day, a number of days in succession. As wastes are gradually cleared, the intestinal environment becomes progressively healthier, and therefore increasingly inhospitable to the microforms that produce acids.

ARE FASTS AND MONO DIETS EFFECTIVE METHODS OF DEACIDIFICATION?

Drainage treatments imposed to remedy ailments other than those due to acidification frequently include measures like fasts or diets restricted to a single food. This is because the restriction of food causes significant amounts of toxins to resurface from the deep tissues, whereupon they can be conducted into the organs of elimination.

These fasts or diets are not the most beneficial treatments for detoxifying the body of acid wastes, however, and therefore cannot generally be recommended. The massive influx of acids they unleash can cause hardships for individuals who suffer from an inability to metabolize acids properly.

Of all the acids that resurface from the deep tissues during a fast, only a small quantity can be eliminated in that form by the organs of elimination. All the others must either be oxidized or buffered. People who have trouble metabolizing acids even at the best of times have little chance of greater success while they fast and these acid wastes appear in greater quantities.

Buffering acids is also problematic. For one reason, the alkaline reserves are generally already depleted; for another, the person on a fast is not ingesting alkaline substances that can support the buffer system. The body therefore must withdraw more alkalines from its reserves without being able to replenish them. This can result in serious mineral depletion.

The situation is different for those who do not have any trouble metabolizing acids. During a fast, their bodies are freed of the necessity of oxidizing acids introduced into the body by food and are able to concentrate on acids already present in the tissues. Because they have a normal capacity to burn off weak acid wastes, they are able to oxidize a good amount; and because they have large alkaline reserves, it is just as easy to buffer acids.

With regard to mono diets, several scenarios are possible. As a rule, mono diets are not beneficial unless they are composed of alkaline foods such as carrots or potatoes, whether the individual has trouble metabolizing acids or not. When a mono diet involves a significant intake of alkaline substances that are not accompanied by acids, these alkaline elements can be fully used to buffer the built-up acid wastes. Furthermore, the energy saved on the digestive level by not having to deal with complicated meals can be utilized to intensify the elimination of acids by the kidneys and sweat glands.

Mono diets composed of acidifying foods, in contrast, are distinctly harmful, because the intake of these foods is not compensated for by alkaline foods. To neutralize these acids—both those that are already built up in the body and those introduced by the mono diet—the body is forced to withdraw what it needs entirely from its reserves without being able to replenish them through new food intake.

Mono diets composed of weak-acid foods—like fruits—are to be strictly avoided by individuals who have trouble metabolizing acids, but are strongly recommended for others because of their ability to oxidize acids. These foods are transformed into alkaline substances that help alkalize the body's internal environment.

This diet is based on alkaline water, green food, and soups and juices made from green vegetables—in other words, a diet that consists only of alkaline foods.

Alkaline water can be either a bottled mineral water from an alkaline spring, or water purified by distillation or reverse osmosis that has had alkaline drops added to raise its pH.

The green-food supplement is mixed with pure water to create a beverage. One teaspoon of green food to every liter of water is the average dose for a delicious alkalizing drink, but the amount of green food can be raised if you prefer a stronger-tasting beverage.

Vegetable juice should be made with an electric (centrifuge) juicer using various green vegetables like cucumbers, cabbage, broccoli, spinach, celery, lettuce, zucchini, peppers, parsley, and so on. Although carrots and beets are not green, they can also be used because they are alkaline vegetables; their natural sugar content gives a more pleasant taste to the juice mixtures. Because vegetable juices are highly concentrated, it is a good idea to dilute them with water before drinking them. If you do not have the proper equipment for juicing vegetables, the juices can be replaced by beverages made from green food. Prepare the soups from these same vegetables and several potatoes, but without salt. Use one to two pounds of vegetables that you let simmer in water until they get tender, then put everything in a blender and make a souplike puree. You can use mild spices such as parsley, rosemary, and laurel. Of course, the vegetables can also be eaten cooked, without being prepared as a soup.

Over the course of the treatment, every day drink around 2 liters of alkaline water, 2 liters of green food beverage, and as much vegetable juice you want. The volume of liquid you drink (which will vary depending on your capacity), in combination with the properties of the vegetables and the green food, stimulates the intestines to work more intensively and evacuate several times a day. If this doesn't happen, take laxative and liver-support preparations to ensure regular elimination of the wastes and acids this diet has flushed out of the internal cellular environment.

Because of the strong purifying effect of this cure on the intestines as well as the kidneys, two to three days on this diet should bring about a good cleansing; but a longer period of a week, for example, will have an even more profound effect on the purification and deacidification of the body.

Here is an example of a typical day's schedule on this cure.

As the body is used to having meals at specific hours of the day, something a bit more solid should be provided at these times: vegetable soup at noon and 6:00, and vegetable juices at 8:00 in the morning and 5:00 in the evening. Consume alkaline water and green-food beverages over the remainder of this period.

7:00–8:00	alkaline water
8:00	green vegetable juice
9:00–11:00	green food beverages and alkaline water
12:00	green vegetable soup
1:00–5:00	green food beverages and alkaline water
5:00	green vegetable juice
6:00	green vegetable soup
7:00–10:00	alkaline water

10

Alkaline Energy Boosters

In addition to taking alkaline supplements to support the body's removal of acid wastes, you may also wish to try energy boosters rich in vitamins and minerals to increase your overall vitality. The most common products of this nature are bee pollen, wheat germ, and brewer's yeast. These products and other energy boosters contain a wide range of nutrients in their natural state, which are very easy for the body to assimilate and represent a sure source of revitalization.

Unfortunately, a number of these products are acidifying and therefore not recommended if you are suffering from any of the disorders due to acidification. Among these are sea buckthorn, which is rich in vitamin C and silica; brewer's yeast, which contains purines, the precursors to uric acid; and bee pollen and, to a lesser extent, royal jelly. It may not be necessary to avoid such products completely, but their use is a delicate matter. It is preferable to use alkaline energy boosters, which include spirulina, blackstrap molasses, ginseng, wheat germ, and halibut liver oil.

The properties, indications, and instructions for using these energy boosters are detailed below. There is no reason whatsoever that you cannot use a supplement and an energy booster at the same time. There is no risk of overdose or an ineffective double application, because the energy boosters are not characterized by their high mineral content but by their high content of vitamins, trace elements, and other nutrients.

Spirulina

Spirulina is an algae that grows in fresh water. It thrives best in alkaline waters with a pH that falls anywhere between 8.5 and 11. The use of spirulina as a food is not of recent origin. Traditionally, various African peoples have eaten it to vary their diet (which is essentially composed of millet). The Aztecs cultivated this algae in their lakes during an earlier era. Harvested with the help of fine-mesh baskets that let the water run out but retained the "green foam," the foam was set out to dry then transported throughout the Aztec empire.

The subject of numerous studies, spirulina is recognized today as an energy booster of the first order. It contains more protein, more beta-carotene (vitamin A), vitamin B_{12}, iron, and gamma-linolenic acid (vitamin F) than any other food known. Its vitamin E content is equal to that of wheat germ, otherwise its most abundant source. Spirulina's concentration of calcium and magnesium is equivalent to that of milk. Furthermore, it contains a complete range of vitamins, minerals, and trace elements.

A third of an ounce (10 g) of spirulina powder is enough to cover the daily need for vitamin B_{12} five times over, four times that for vitamin A, 83 percent of the daily requirement for iron, 30 percent of vitamin B_2, and 25 percent of vitamin B_1.

Spirulina is particularly recommended for fatigue, anemia, eyesight problems, menstrual problems, and skin disorders. In addition, it helps strengthen the immune system and facilitates the elimination of toxins that have collected inside the body.

It comes in the form of a deep-green powder with a faint aroma, and also in tablets or capsules.

When combined with foods, spirulina turns them all green. For this reason it is most often used in tablet or capsule form for therapies intended to boost the body's vitality. A tablet generally contains 500 mg of spirulina. The recommended daily dosage for intensive treatments is $1/3$ ounce (10 g), which corresponds to 20 tablets, or a heaping tablespoon of powder. For maintenance therapies or when there are no urgent health issues, the doses can easily be divided into halves or thirds. Spirulina tablets should be taken with water three times a day before meals; the powder is usually eaten in combination with food.

Blackstrap Molasses

Blackstrap molasses is a byproduct of the pressing of sugar cane. It is a sugar-rich sap that has a high content of minerals, vitamins, and trace elements.

To separate the sugar from the rest of the elements, the sap is heated in a vat. The heat causes the sugar to crystallize; the crystals sink to the bottom of the vat and are harvested as whole or natural sugar. What remains on the top is a thick syrup containing the essential nutrients of the sugar cane.

Thus, whole sugar obtained through this process is not as whole as it could be. In fact, true whole sugar contains black-strap molasses and sugar. It is produced without cooking by exposing sugar cane sap to the sun in large flat tubs so the liquid content evaporates.

Although it still contains sugar, blackstrap molasses is primarily used for its high mineral content. Three and a half ounces (100 g) of blackstrap molasses contains 1,900 to 3,300 mg of potassium, 800 to 1,400 mg of calcium, 300 to 400 mg of magnesium, 15 to 28 mg of iron, and so on. Its potassium content is higher, gram for gram, than that of soy, brewer's yeast, vegetables, or fruits, all foods considered the most important sources of potassium.

Blackstrap molasses is as rich in magnesium as wheat germ, almonds, figs, and dates, which are all generally recommended as sources of this important mineral.

137

Likewise, iron is present in higher levels in blackstrap molasses than in liver, spinach, apricots, or eggs.

Blackstrap molasses is especially recommended for anemia, cramps, edema, rheumatism, insomnia, and stress.

It is available in liquid or solid (flake) form. It has a slightly sugary flavor with a pronounced taste of sugar cane.

The daily dose is 2 to 3 full teaspoons of liquid, or 1 to 2 tablespoons of the flakes. It can be eaten at one time or divided into 3 daily doses in the form of a hot or cold drink. For a hot beverage, the blackstrap molasses is blended directly with water; for a cold drink, it must first be dissolved in hot water before cold water is added.

It is advisable to drink this mixture slowly and hold it in the mouth long enough to mix it with a good amount of saliva in order to avoid bloating and flatulence.

Blackstrap molasses treatments generally last 1 to 2 months, but can be extended if necessary.

Ginseng

Ginseng is a plant native to the Far East that grows in the underbrush of woods and forests. It has been recognized and used for more than four thousand years for its curative and energy-boosting properties. At one time it was so esteemed it cost its own weight in gold.

The root is the part of the plant that is utilized. Over the course of its growth the root acquires enormous proportions in comparison with the root-to-stem proportion of most other plants. The ginseng root can grow to 4 feet in length and 4 inches in width, whereas the stem reaches a height of only 12 to 32 inches. The root must be at least six or seven years old before it is harvested. The wealth of ginseng's properties can be gauged from the exhaustion of the soil it grows in: after harvest, the ground must be left fallow for twelve years before it can again be used.

Ginseng root is characterized primarily by its high content of B vitamins, but it also contains vitamins A, C, D, and E, as well as an assortment of minerals and trace elements. Its healing properties appear to derive from a substance called ginsenoid. Preparations with a ginseng base should contain at least 6 percent of this substance.

There are many uses for ginseng, among them treating states of exhaustion and chronic fatigue, degenerative illnesses, depression, nervous system disorders, diabetes, and stress, as well as problems with liver function, memory, and convalescence.

In the past, ginseng treatments simply consisted of eating a small piece of the root on a daily basis. Today, liquid ginseng extract is the preferred method of use because it provides a concentrated form of the plant's active principles. The dosage level should be specified by the extract's manufacturer. Usually the extract comes with a small spoon made to hold the recommended dosage.

Treatments can extend from four to six weeks and can be repeated as needed over the year.

Wheat Germ Sprouts

The germ is the most nutritious part of the wheat seed. The germ contains in concentrated form the major portion of the nutrients necessary for the plant's future growth: amino acids, essential fatty acids, numerous minerals, trace elements, all the B vitamins, and a high concentration of vitamin E. This exceptional nutrient content is what permits the plant to grow so explosively during its first days of life.

Surprisingly, the growth of the germ does not reduce its reserves but increases them. This makes the wheat germ even richer than it was before germination. Thanks to enzymes, new nutrients are produced. For $3^1/2$ ounces (100 g) of wheat germ sprouts, the level of calcium rises from 45 to 71 mg, and that of magnesium from 133 to 342 mg. Vitamin content increases 20 percent for vitamin B_1, 45 percent for vitamin B_5, 200 percent for vitamin B_6, 225 percent for the proto-vitamin A, 300 percent for vitamin E, and 500 percent for vitamin C.

To sprout wheat, place the grains in a glass of water for twelve hours, then spread them on a plate near a window (for the light) and moisten them twice a day. Within three or four days the germ will sprout. It first appears as a white tip, then lengthens into a short stem that gradually changes color from white to green.

Wheat germ sprouts can be eaten when the sprout has reached a length of $^1/10$ to $^1/5$ inch (3 to 5 mm). At this stage it is still white. The germ is eaten with the grain and the tiny roots that have formed. It has a pleasant flavor and is an especially good addition to salads.

To have a daily supply of germinated wheat sprouts, start a new batch every day on a plate. Sprout trays with several levels are available commercially; they can replace plates and are much more convenient to use.

In addition to its energy-boosting properties, wheat germ is indicated for hypotension, depression, a tendency toward thrombosis (blood clots), and painful or irregular menstrual periods.

The daily dose is a level tablespoon of dried wheat seeds. Because of the sprouts' extremely revitalizing properties, an overdose can lead to a state of physical or psychic excitation. Sprouted wheat germ is therefore not recommended for those with high blood pressure, and its consumption in the evening is not advised. The daily dose can be taken at one time, either with breakfast or lunch.

The treatment generally lasts two to three weeks, and can be repeated as needed.

Halibut Liver Oil

Halibut is a fish found in the waters of the North Atlantic whose liver contains an oil that is quite rich in vitamin D. It contains 2 to 3 million international units (IU) of vitamin D per $3^{1}/2$ ounces (100 g), whereas the other foods with the highest vitamin D content—butter, eggs, and cheese—have only 200 IU per 7 ounces (200 g).

Vitamin D not only encourages the absorption of calcium on the intestinal level, but it also contributes to maintaining a constant level of blood calcium, thus allowing the cells access to calcium at all times. Vitamin D also promotes the ability of calcium to remain fixed to the skeletal structure, therefore conferring solidity to the bones. Both the bloodstream and the skeleton are two important reserves from which the body can withdraw calcium in its fight against acidification.

Halibut liver oil is especially recommended for people suffering from acidification, because it prevents the decalcification of the skeleton due to acidity, as well as that caused by a deficiency in vitamin D.

In addition to vitamin D, halibut liver oil contains large quantities of vitamin A, whose well-known role in the optimal health of the eyes and skin is supplemented by its action on the skeleton. As a co-factor of vitamin D, vitamin A contributes to the formation of bones and to calcium retention.

Halibut liver oil is generally recommended during the winter, because this is the season that receives the least sunlight. The sun plays a significant role in the calcification of the skeleton, as the skin can manufacture vitamin D when it is exposed to sunlight.

This oil can treat rickets, decalcification problems, bone fractures, osteoporosis, and a tendency to dental cavities. It is also recommended for the growing years and for menopause.

Today the oil is sold in capsules to be swallowed with water. As vitamin D is a lipid-soluble vitamin, it is better digested and assimilated by the body if it is taken in the middle of a meal, preferably one that contains some fatty foods.

It is important to follow the manufacturer's dosage instructions, because an overdose of vitamin D can be harmful to a person's health.

These treatments can extend for two to three months. Acidified individuals do not need to wait for winter to begin their treatment, but can start it whenever they please. Subsequently, the treatment should be repeated on a yearly basis during the cold months.

Sicknesses do not appear suddenly and for no reason; they are the result of causes that need to be dealt with in order for the sickness to disappear. The cause of acid problems in the body lies in the way people eat and live. The information in this book shows you how to modify these factors in order to be healthy again. I wish readers every success in your quest for good health.

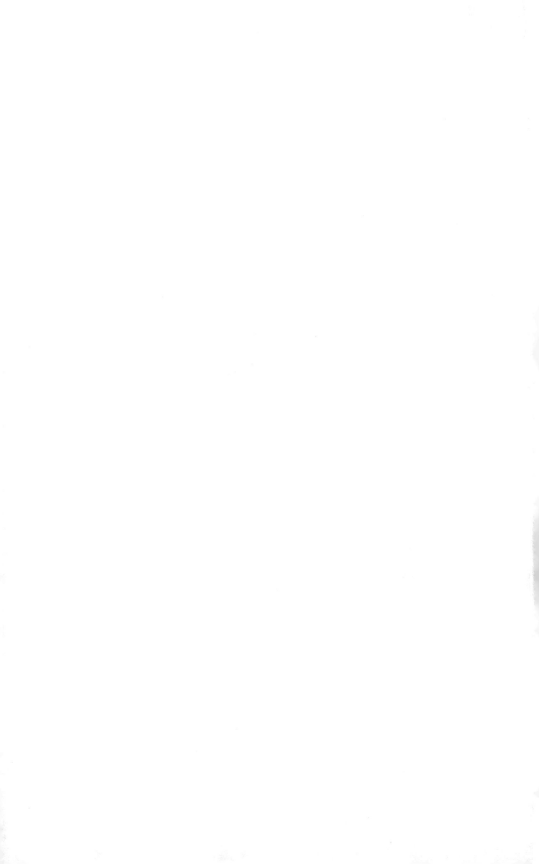

CPSIA information can be obtained
at www.ICGtesting.com
Printed in the USA
LVHW050501220221
679517LV00017B/931